# GLENN'S GAMES

## GLENN SEYMOUR

authorHOUSE®

*AuthorHouse™*
*1663 Liberty Drive*
*Bloomington, IN 47403*
*www.authorhouse.com*
*Phone: 1-800-839-8640*

*Published by AuthorHouse 11/05/2013*

*ISBN: 978-1-4918-3251-6 (sc)*
*ISBN: 978-1-4918-3250-9 (e)*

*Library of Congress Control Number: 2013919356*

In loving memory of our Dad

Glenn Seymour

Harold
Maurice
Marjorie
Kenny
Maxine (Teenie)
Donna Jeane
Lonnie
Bonnie

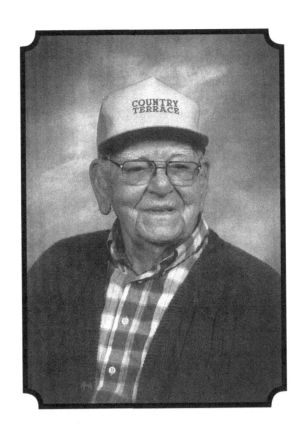

Glenn Seymour always led an active life with his large family, his work delivering mail, his garden and other hobbies. When he moved to Country Terrace Senior Living Apartments at the age of 90 his eyesight was failing and walking was growing more difficult. Glenn believed in keeping as active as possible so he joined the exercise class and participated in all of the activities Country Terrace offered. He was delighted in making up these games to keep his own mind active and to share with the other residents. He was still making up games when he passed away a few months before his 99th birthday. Enjoy these games and see if your mind is as sharp as Glenn's was.

# GLENN'S BOOK OF GAMES
## CREATED BY GLENN SEYMOUR

## INDEX

# ANIMALS

# BIRDS
## CREATED BY GLENN SEYMOUR

1.  Bird of peace and love _____

2.  Bird used to detect gas in mines_____

3.  Smallest singing bird _____

4.  Bird that lives on nectar _____

5.  The honking bird _____

6.  Singing bird kept in the house _____

7.  Taken far away, set free, will return home _____

8.  Quacking bird _____

9.  Bird that carries messages _____

10. Birds that coo _____

11. Bird that its bill holds more than its belly _____

12. Has a ring around its neck _____

13. Another name of quail _____

14. Wise bird _____

15. Only bird that can fly backwards _____

16. Bird catches prey in flight with its claws _____

17. Prefers to nest in hedge about 4" above ground_____

18. Largest bird _____

19. Bird that can form large fantail _____

20. Sit quietly close together on a perch_____

21. We watch for in the early spring_____

22. Bird with word English in its name _____

23. Two talking birds _____

24. Comes to feeder when all others leave _____

25. Bright red bird _____

26. Bird that likes an apartment house_____

27. Bird often mounted as a trophy _____

28. Web footed birds _____

29. A bird that will follow ships _____

30. Speaks its name usually at dusk _____

31. Bird with long neck _____

32. Small bird likes a little house _____

33. Night hunter_____

34. Bird that lays bright blue eggs _____

35. Extinct bird _____

36. United States bird_____

37. Hunts insects around bark of tree _____

38. Bird eats mostly rodents_____

39. Wild bird for Thanksgiving _____

40. Bird that imitates several birds_____

41. A common wild duck_____

42. Likes to bore holes in trees _____

43. Two birds that live in a barn_____

44. Produces down feathers for pillows _____

45. Flies at dusk, feeds on mosquitoes & insects _____

46. Has ears on top of his head like a cat _____

47. Birds with the tail coat _____

48. Small bird that will run along side of car _____

# BIRDS
## CREATED BY GLENN SEYMOUR

1.  Bird of peace and love.................................................................... dove

2.  Bird used to detect gas in mines.................................................canary

3.  Smallest singing bird.................................................................wren

4.  Bird that lives on nectar.........................................................hummingbird

5.  The honking bird.................................................................. goose

6.  Singing bird kept in the house..................................................canary

7.  Taken far away, set free, will return home...............................homing pigeon

8.  Quacking bird........................................................................duck

9.  Bird that carries messages ....................................................carrier pigeon

10. Birds that coo.....................................................................dove - pigeon

11. Bird that its bill holds more than its belly...............................pelican

12. Has a ring around its neck ......................................... ring neck pheasant

13. Another name of quail............................................... bob white

14. Wise bird ............................................................................. owl

15. Only bird that can fly backwards...............................................hummingbird

16. Bird catches prey in flight with its claws ............................... hawk

17. Prefers to nest in hedge about 4" above ground........................ brown thrush

18. Largest bird ............................................................... ostrich

19. Bird that can form large fantail..............................................peacock

20. Sit quietly close together on a perch ................................... love birds

21. We watch for in the early spring............................................robin

22. Bird with word English in its name ...................................... English sparrow

23. Two talking birds................................................... parrot - mime bird

24. Comes to feeder when all others leave .................................blue jay

25. Bright red bird ............................................................ cardinal

26. Bird that likes an apartment house ................................... martin

27. Bird often mounted as a trophy...............................................pheasant

28. Web footed bird ....................................................................duck - goose - swan

29. A bird that will follow ships ........................................................ sea gull

30. Speaks its name usually at dusk ................................................whippoorwill

31. Bird with long neck .........................................................................crane

32. Small bird likes a little house ...........................................................wren

33. Night hunter ...................................................................................... owl

34. Bird that lays bright blue eggs .......................................................robin

35. Extinct bird .......................................................................................dodo

36. United States bird .........................................................................eagle

37. Hunts insects around bark of tree ...........................................chickadee

38. Bird eats mostly rodents ................................................................. owl

39. Wild bird for Thanksgiving......................................................... turkey

40. Bird that imitates several birds .............................................mocking bird

41. A common wild duck ...................................................................mallard

42. Likes to bore holes in trees........................................................woodpecker

43. Two birds that live in a barn ..................................... barn owl - barn swallow

44. Produces down feathers for pillows......................................... goose

45. Flies at dusk, feeds on mosquitoes & insects .................................. swallow

46. Has ears on top of his head like a cat....................................... owl

47. Birds with the tail coat...................................................................penguin

48. Small bird that will run along side of car ........................................ swallow

# ANIMALS
## CREATED BY GLENN SEYMOUR

1.   Stubborn animal _____

2.   Dumb animal _____

3.   Sly animal _____

4.   Animal used to hard work_____

5.   Three animals used for meat _____

6.   Animal with a goatee_____

7.   Gentle as a _____

8.   Animal called Smokey the_____

9.   Animal kept for their milk _____

10.  Animal that has a pouch _____

11.  Animal that never forgets _____

12.  Animal that produces pork _____

13.  Farm animal with horns _____

14.  Animal that has a long neck _____

15.  Animal that roars _____

16.  Animal that laughs _____

17.  Animal that likes honey _____

18.  A little cuddly bear _____

19.  A small horse_____

20.  Animal that has spots _____

21.  Has it own powder puff_____

22.  Man's best friend _____

23.  Cuts trees, builds dams _____

24.  Big burly animal that roamed the plains years ago _____

25.  Used to drive game out of burrows _____

26.  Animal with humps_____

27.  Animals with antlers _____

28.  Animal plays dead when molested _____

11

29. Defends itself with needles _____

30. Very playful in water _____

31. Very fast runner _____

32. Defends itself with foul odor _____

33. Likes to stay at night in tree tops _____

34. Forecasts length of winter _____

35. A good mouser _____

36. Cat with very short tail _____

37. Hibernates in winter _____

38. Animal with stripes _____

39. Two animals with tusks _____

40. Two animals that can bark _____

41. Three animals that howl _____

42. Two animals that can walk upright _____

43. Valuable fur _____

44. Two animals that hop _____

45. Animal that likes to wash its food _____

46. Two animals that have a mane _____

47. Pack animal used on trails _____

48. Animal that has nine lives _____

49. Animal that can hang by its tail _____

50. Animal that roots in the soil _____

51. Animal you count to get to sleep _____

52. Animal that chews its cud _____

53. Two animals that are scavengers _____

54. Animals that hunt in packs _____

55. Animal with more than one stomach _____

56. Animal that is a great climber _____

57. Animal that lives on bamboo _____

58. Animal that is transportation in the desert _____

# ANIMALS
## CREATED BY GLENN SEYMOUR

1.  Stubborn animal ................................................................mule

2.  Dumb animal .................................................................... ox

3.  Sly animal ......................................................................fox

4.  Animal used to hard work ...................................... draft horse

5.  Three animals used for meat.........................cow - hog - sheep

6.  Animal with a goatee ........................................................goat

7.  Gentle as a .....................................................................lamb

8.  Animal called Smokey the ................................................bear

9.  Animal kept for their milk ............................................... cow

10.  Animal that has a pouch.............................................kangaroo

11.  Animal that never forgets............................................ elephant

12.  Animal that produces pork ................................................pig

13.  Farm animal with horns ................................................. cow

14.  Animal that has a long neck............................................ giraffe

15.  Animal that roars .............................................................lion

16.  Animal that laughs ........................................................hyena

17.  Animal that likes honey..................................................bear

18.  A little cuddly bear .......................................................koala

19.  A small horse ................................................................pony

20.  Animal that has spots ..................................................leopard

21.  Has it own powder puff .................................................rabbit

22.  Man's best friend.............................................................dog

23.  Cuts trees, builds dams.................................................beaver

24.  Big burly animal that roamed the plains years ago...........buffalo

25.  Used to drive game out of burrows.................................ferret

26.  Animal with humps .......................................................camel

27.  Animals with antlers ......................................................deer

28.  Animal plays dead when molested ...............................possum

29. Defends itself with needles .................................................................porcupine

30. Very playful in water ............................................................................. otter

31. Very fast runner ....................................................................................cheetah

32. Defends itself with foul odor .................................................................skunk

33. Likes to stay at night in tree tops ...................................................... raccoon

34. Forecasts length of winter .................................................................groundhog

35. A good mouser ...................................................................................... cat

36. Cat with a very short tail ......................................................................lynx

37. Hibernates in winter ..............................................................................bear

38. Animal with stripes ...............................................................................zebra

39. Two animals with tusks ........................................... elephant - wild boar

40. Two animals that can bark .............................................................dog - coyote

41. Three animals that howl ......................................................dog - wolf - coyote

42. Two animals that can walk upright ...............................................bear - monkey

43. Valuable fur ............................................................ ermine - mink - sable

44. Two animals that hop ...................................................... rabbit - kangaroo

45. Animal that likes to wash its food .................................................. raccoon

46. Two animals that have a mane .................................................. horse - lion

47. Pack animal used on trails ....................................................... burro

48. Animal that has nine lives ........................................................... cat

49. Animal that can hang by its tail ............................................... monkey

50. Animal that roots in the soil ..................................................... hog

51. Animal you count to get to sleep ............................................... sheep

52. Animal that chews its cud ......................................................... cow

53. Two animals that are scavengers ...................................... possum - hyena

54. Animals that hunt in packs .......................... wolves - coyotes - wild hogs

55. Animal with more than one stomach ................................................ camel

56. Animal that is a great climber ...........................................mountain goat

57. Animal that lives on bamboo.............................................................panda

58. Animal that is transportation in the desert ................................... camel

# DOWN ON THE FARM
CREATED BY GLENN SEYMOUR

1. What is a female bovine? _____

2. What is a male bovine? _____

3. What is a baby bovine? _____

4. What is a young female bovine? _____

5. What is a group of cows? _____

6. A man that cares for cattle is? _____

7. What is cow meat? _____

8. What is an equine? _____

9. What is a female horse? _____

10. What is a male horse? _____

11. What is a baby horse? _____

12. What is a home for a horse? _____

13. What is a horse rider? _____

14. What are swine? _____

15. What is a female hog? _____

16. What is a male hog? _____

17. What is a baby hog? _____

18. What is a home for a pig? _____

19. What is a group of pigs? _____

20. What is hog meat? _____

21. What is a female sheep? _____

22. What is a male sheep? _____

23. What is a baby sheep? _____

24. What is a group of sheep? _____

25. What is sheep meat? _____

26. Who takes care of sheep? _____

27. What is a male goat? _____

28. What is a female goat? _____

29. What is a baby goat? _____

30. What is the saying goats eat? _____

31. What is a male turkey? _____

32. What is a female turkey? _____

33. What is a baby turkey? _____

34. What is turkey day? _____

35. What is a female rabbit? _____

36. What is a male rabbit? _____

37. What is a baby rabbit? _____

38. Where do rabbits live? _____

39. To what breed do rabbits belong? _____

40. How should you carry a rabbit? _____

41. What is a female duck? _____

42. What is a male duck? _____

43. What is a baby duck? _____

44. What is a female goose? _____

45. What is a male goose? _____

46. What is a baby goose? _____

47. What is a group of geese or ducks? _____

48. Another name for all birds is? _____

# DOWN ON THE FARM
## CREATED BY GLENN SEYMOUR

1.   What is a female bovine? ...................................................................... cow

2.   What is a male bovine? ...........................................................................bull

3.   What is a baby bovine? ........................................................................... calf

4.   What is a young female bovine? .......................................................... heifer

5.   What is a group of cows? ...................................................................... herd

6.   A man that cares for cattle is? ..........................................................cowboy

7.   What is cow meat? ..................................................................................beef

8.   What is an equine? ...............................................................................horse

9.   What is a female horse? .......................................................................mare

10.  What is a male horse? ........................................................................stallion

11.  What is a baby horse? ...........................................................................foal

12.  What is a home for a horse? .................................................................. stall

13.  What is a horse rider? ........................................................................jockey

14 -.  What are swine? ...................................................................................hogs

15.  What is a female hog? ...........................................................................sow

16.  What is a male hog? ............................................................................ boar

17.  What is a baby hog? ..............................................................................pig

18.  What is a home for a pig? .................................................................... sty

19.  What is a group of pigs? .....................................................................litter

20.  What is hog meat? ...............................................................................pork

21.  What is a female sheep? .......................................................................ewe

22.  What is a male sheep? ..........................................................................ram

23.  What is a baby sheep? .........................................................................lamb

24.  What is a group of sheep? ...................................................................flock

25.  What is sheep meat? ........................................................................ mutton

26.  Who takes care of sheep? ...............................................................Sheppard

27. What is a male goat? ....................................................................................buck

28. What is a female goat? ................................................................................ nanny

29. What is a baby goat? ......................................................................................kid

30. What is the saying goats eat? ...................................................................tincans

31. What is a male turkey? ................................................................................. tom

32. What is a female turkey? ...............................................................................hen

33. What is a baby turkey? ............................................................................. poult

34. What is turkey day? ......................................................................... Thanksgiving

35. What is a female rabbit? ...............................................................................doe

36. What is a male rabbit? ..................................................................................buck

37. What is a baby rabbit? ............................................................................. bunny

38. Where do rabbits live? ............................................................................. hutch

39. To what breed do rabbits belong? ...............................................................hare

40. How should you carry a rabbit? ...........................................by fur above the shoulder

41. What is a female duck? .......................................................................... hen - goose

42. What is a male duck? ..................................................................................drake

43. What is a baby duck? ............................................................................. duckling

44. What is a female goose? ........................................................................ hen - goose

45. What is a male goose? .............................................................................. gander

46. What is a baby goose? ...............................................................................gosling

47. What is a group of geese or ducks? ............................................................flock

48. Another name for all birds is? ....................................................................fowl

# ANIMAL NAMES
## CREATED BY GLENN SEYMOUR

1. Kermit _____
2. Cupid _____
3. Perry Winkle _____
4. Elsie _____
5. Flower _____
6. Dumbo _____
7. Lassie _____
8. Silver _____
9. Bambi _____
10. Rudolph _____
11. Mr. Ed _____
12. Mickey _____
13. Porky _____
14. Comet _____
15. Felix _____
16. Minnie _____
17. Harvey _____
18. Donald _____
19. Chubby _____
20. Burr _____
21. Jiminey _____
22. Arnold _____
23. Flipper _____
24. Dasher _____
25. Alvin _____
26. Thumper _____
27. Eager _____
28. Black Beauty _____
29. Vixon _____
30. Polly _____
31. Gentle Ben _____
32. Trigger _____
33. Henny Penny _____
34. Woody _____
35. Garfield _____
36. Flicka _____
37. Benji _____
38. Sly old _____
39. Wise old _____
40. Peter _____
41. Rin Tin Tin _____
42. King Kong _____
43. Old Yeller _____
44. Smokey _____
45. Sylvester _____
46. Dancer _____
47. Miss _____
48. Leo _____
49. Blitzen _____
50. Tony _____
51. Fuzzy Wuzzy _____
52. Robin Red Breast _____

# ANIMAL NAMES
## CREATED BY GLENN SEYMOUR

1. Kermit.................................frog
2. Cupid.................................deer
3. Perry Winkle.....................moose
4. Elsie.................................cow
5. Flower.............................skunk
6. Dumbo.........................elephant
7. Lassie...............................dog
8. Silver..............................horse
9. Bambi.............................fawn
10. Rudolph............red nose reindeer
11. Mr. Ed............................horse
12. Mickey..........................Mouse
13. Porky................................pig
14. Comet.............................deer
15. Felix................................cat
16. Minnie...........................mouse
17. Harvey...........................rabbit
18. Donald.............................duck
19. Chubby...........................bear
20. Burr..............................rabbit
21. Jiminey.........................cricket
22. Arnold..............................pig
23. Flipper..........................dolphin
24. Dasher............................deer
25. Alvin...........................chipmunk
26. Thumper..........................bunny
27. Eager............................beaver
28. Black Beauty....................horse
29. Vixon..............................deer
30. Polly.............................parrot
31. Gentle Ben........................bear
32. Trigger...........................horse
33. Henny Penny.......................hen
34. Woody.......................woodpecker
35. Garfield...........................cat
36. Flicka............................horse
37. Benji...............................dog
38. Sly old.............................fox
39. Wise old...........................owl
40. Peter.............................rabbit
41. Rin Tin Tin.........................dog
42. King Kong..........................ape
43. Old Yeller..........................dog
44. Smokey............................bear
45. Sylvester...........................cat
46. Dancer.............................deer
47. Miss..............................piggy
48. Leo................................lion
49. Blitzen.............................deer
50. Tony..............................tiger
51. Fuzzy Wuzzy.......................bear
52. Robin Red Breast..................bird

# AROUND THE HOUSE

# GROCERY STORE
CREATED BY GLENN SEYMOUR

1. Iceberg _____

2. Purple Top _____

3. Vidalia _____

4. Icicle _____

5. Honeydew _____

6. Alberta _____

7. Winesap _____

8. Naval _____

9. Nancy Hall _____

10. Blue Gage _____

11. Burpless _____

12. Beef Steak _____

13. Russet _____

14. Strawberry _____

15. BoPeep _____

16. Longhorn _____

17. Imperial _____

18. Cottage _____

19. Meadow Gold _____

20. Whipping _____

21. Sunbeam _____

22. Hamburger _____

23. Ritz _____

24. Premium _____

25. Vanilla _____

26. Whole Kernel _____

27. Jif _____

28. Osage _____

29. Folgers _____

30. Campbell _____

31. Lipton _____

32. Vanity Fair _____

33. Redenbocker _____

34. Bayer _____

35. Colgate _____

36. Scope _____

37. Birds Eye _____

38. Pringles _____

# GROCERY STORE
### CREATED BY GLENN SEYMOUR

1. Iceberg............................lettuce
2. Purple Top ..........................turnip
3. Vidalia ............................onion
4. Icicle ............................radish
5. Honeydew.......................melon
6. Alberta ..........................peach
7. Winesap ........................apple
8. Naval............................orange
9. Nancy Hall.................. sweet potato
10. Blue Gage......................plum
11. Burpless........................cucumber
12. Beef steak.....................tomato
13. Russet ..........................potato
14. Strawberry.....................rhubarb
15. BoPeep ..........................ammonia
16. Longhorn.......................cheese
17. Imperial.........................oleo
18. Cottage.........................cheese
19. Meadow Gold....................milk

20. Whipping.......................cream
21. Sunbeam ........................bread
22. Hamburger .......................buns
23. Ritz..........................crackers
24. Premium .......................crackers
25. Vanilla .........................wafers
26. Whole kernel......................corn
27. Jif........................peanut butter
28. Osage ..........................peaches
29. Forgers........................coffee
30. Campbell........................soup
31. Lipton .............................tea
32. Vanity Fair .....................napkins
33. Redenbocker.......................popcorn
34. Bayer...........................aspirin
35. Colgate ........................tooth paste
36. Scope ........................mouthwash
37. Birds Eye ......................frozen food
38. Pringles .....................potato chips

# OLD CARS
## CREATED BY GLENN SEYMOUR

1.   Name for an old car _____

2.   An old banged up car _____

3.   That rubber tube on the drivers side _____

4.   Some early cars were not gas but _____

5.   Hand lever at drivers side _____

6.   Two foot pedals _____

7.   In case of rain how did we close the car _____

8.   What was the old open car _____

9.   What was the open end seater _____

10.  If you put the top down you had a _____

11.  Heater in old car _____

12.  How was foot warmer prepared _____

13.  What did you step onto get in or out _____

14.  Where was the gas tank _____

15.  What created spark _____

16.  How did you start an early car _____

17.  What composed a seat _____

18.  How many cylinders did it have _____

19.  What was the first trunk _____

20.  Early tires had _____

21.  What was different about the windshield _____

22.  What was a car with glass windows called _____

23.  What was a one seated closed car called _____

24.  Trunk opened to make a _____

25.  Put on tires when it is snowing _____

26.  Older cars were what color _____

# OLD CARS
## CREATED BY GLENN SEYMOUR

1.  Name for an old car..........................................................Jitney-Fliver-Jalopy

2.  An old banged up car......................................................................Clunker

3.  That rubber tube on the drivers side..............................................Horn

4.  Some early cars were not gas but....................................................Electric

5.  Hand lever at drivers side.................................................Emergency Brake

6.  Two foot pedals.....................................................................Clutch - Brake

7.  In case of rain how did we close the car..............................Side Curtains

8.  What was the old open car............................................................Touring Car

9.  What was the open end seater.........................................................Roadster

10. If you put the top down you had a............................Sports Roadster

11. Heater in old car.................................laprobe - bricks or stone foot warmer

12. How was foot warmer prepared...................preheated in oven or wrapped in wood

13. What did you step onto get in or out.......................... Running Board

14. Where was the gas tank.........................under front seat - outside above dash

15. What created spark...............................................................Magneto Coils

16. How did you start an early car........................................................ Crank

17. What composed a seat..............................Coil springs - Imitation Leather

18. How many cylinders did it have...................................................Four

19. What was the first trunk.............................................Metal box on the back

20. Early tires had ...........................................................................Inner Tube

21. What was different about the windsheild ...........................It could be turned down

22. What was a car with glass windows called........................................Sedan

23. What was a one seated closed car.....................................................Coupe

24. Trunk opened to make a ........................................................Rumble Seat

25. Put on tires when it is snowing....................................................Chains

26. Older cars were what color ...............................................................Black

# NEWER CARS
## CREATED BY GLENN SEYMOUR

1.   If you wish to maintain one speed _____

2.   Forget to turn off lights _____

3.   Leave keys in ignition _____

4.   Get too warm you turn on_____

5.   To tell the time you have a_____

6.   To keep you up on the news you have a _____

7.   Seat needs adjusting you have _____

8.   If you have a flat tire you have an _____

9.   Windshield is dirty you have_____

10.  Your windows and doors locks are _____

11.   In case of snow and ice you have _____

12.  Two types of transmissions are _____

13.  Present tires do not have _____

14.  You can get your new in what color _____

15.  Can you name three car makers _____

16.  What is a car without a metal top _____

# NEWER CARS
## CREATED BY GLENN SEYMOUR

1. If you wish to maintain one speed .................................................................. Speed control

2. Forget to turn off lights................................................................................. Buzzer sounds

3. Leave keys in ignition ..................................................................................... Buzzer sounds

4. Get too warm you turn on .............................................................................. Air conditioner

5. To tell the time you have a.............................................................................. Clock on the dash

6. To keep you up on the news you have a ....................................................... Radio

7. Seat needs adjusting you have ....................................................................... Electric adjustable Seats

8. If you have a flat tire you have an ................................................................. Inflated tire in the trunk

9. Windshield is dirty you have .......................................................................... Electric windshield washers

10. Your windows and doors locks are .............................................................. Electrically controlled

11. In case of snow and ice you have.................................................................. Snow tires

12. Two types of transmissions are...................................................................... Automatic - shift

13. Present tires do not have ................................................................................ Tubes

14. You can get your new in what color............................................................... Different

15. Can you name three car makers..................................................................... Ford-Chevrolet-Honda

16. What is a car without a metal top .................................................................. Convertible

# HARDWARE
### CREATED BY GLENN SEYMOUR

1. Cutting tool _____

2. Nail driver _____

3. Measuring device _____

4. What you drive with a hammer_____

5. Fasten things together _____

6. Carry to see things in the dark _____

7. Paint applier _____

8. Garden chopper _____

9. Lawn seats _____

10. Flashlight power _____

11. Garden sprinkler_____

12. Grass clippers _____

13. Makes grass grow _____

14. Stir garden soil _____

15. A quick cooker _____

16. Copper clad_____

17. Pulverizer _____

18. Illuminators_____

19. Floor swaps _____

20. An absorber_____

21. Keeps doors closed _____

22. Keeps flies out _____

23. To fill nail holes _____

24. To hang doors _____

25. Trim shrubbery_____

26. To dig a hole _____

27. To scoop grain _____

28. Loosen a bolt _____

29. Food heat detector _____

30. Stretch dough _____

31. Stirrer _____

32. Frying pan _____

33. Used to cut metal _____

34. Wiring for a lamp _____

35. Used to cut cloth _____

36. Used for pressing _____

37. Outside clothes dryer _____

38. Keeps clothes on line _____

39. To make small holes _____

40. Turn water on & off _____

41. Something in links _____

42. Fasten fence to post _____

# HARDWARE
## CREATED BY GLENN SEYMOUR

1. Cutting tool ................................................................ axe    saw    knife

2. Nail driver ...........................................................................hammer

3. Measuring device ..............................tape measure   yard stick   ruler

4. What you drive with a hammer............................................. nails

5. Fasten things together...........................................................bolts

6. Carry to see things in the dark ..................................... flashlight

7. Paint applier ......................................................brush   roller

8. Garden chopper ....................................................................hoe

9. Lawn seats ......................................... chairs    swings    gliders

10. Flashlight power ........................................................batteries

11. Garden sprinkler ............................................................ hose

12. Grass clippers........................................................lawn mower

13. Makes grass grow ................................................... fertilizer

14. Stir garden soil ............................................................. tiller

15. A quick cooker............................................pressure cooker

16. Copper clad ..............................................................pots    pans

17. Pulverizer ............................................................ food grinder

18. Illuminators.........................................................light bulbs

19. Floor swaps......................................................... mop

20. An absorber.............................................................. sponge

21. Keeps doors closed..................................................latch   lock

22. Keeps flies out ..................................................screens

23. To fill nail holes............................................................ putty

24. To hang doors ....................................................hinge

25. Trim shrubbery...........................................................clippers

26. To dig a hole................................................................ spade

27. To scoop grain ................................................................................................ shovel

28. Loosen a bolt................................................................................................ wrench

29. Food heat detector........................................................................... thermometer

30. Stretch dough.................................................................................... rolling pin

31. Stirrer .......................................................................................... electric mixer

32. Frying pan ............................................................................................ skillet

33. Used to cut metal.............................................................................. tin snips

34. Wiring for a lamp ........................................................................electric cord

35. Used to cut cloth............................................................................... scissors

36. Used for pressing ..................................................................................... iron

37. Outside clothes dryer........................................................................clothesline

38. Keeps clothes on line........................................................................clothespins

39. To make small holes ................................................................................ drill

40. Turn water on & off................................................................................faucet

41. Something in links ................................................................................chain

42. Fasten fence to post.............................................................................staples

# TAXES
CREATED BY GLENN SEYMOUR

1. Tax on earnings _____

2. Tax on food, clothing _____

3. Tax taken out of salary _____

4. Tax on gasoline _____

5. Tax paid on farm or home _____

6. Tax paid on receipt of a large estate _____

7. Tax on large amounts given a person _____

8. Tax some cities charge on cars _____

9. Tax on alcohol _____

10. Tax on jewelry _____

11. Tax on profits on investments _____

12. Tax on gas, water, lights _____

13. Things not taxed _____

14. Tax filing date _____

15. Forecasting what your taxes will be _____

16. How often are estimated taxes paid _____

17. Charges for parking _____

18. Charges on highways and bridges _____

19. Costs added for late payment of taxes _____

20. Taxes not paid on time _____

21. A contract is an _____

22. Anything put up to secure a loan _____

23. Owner of rental property _____

24. Renter of property _____

25. Money paid to live in someone's house _____

26. Agreement between owner and renter _____

27. Papers showing ownership and title _____

28. Papers showing location, description, history of property _____

29. Money loaned to purchase property _____

30. Money charges for the use of money _____

31. A financial claim fixed against property _____

32. Money charged to place values on property for a loan _____

33. Two main forms of farm rent _____

34. Rent for boarding a pasture _____

35. A fee paid to bind a contract for a time _____

36. Tax deduction on your home _____

# TAXES
## CREATED BY GLENN SEYMOUR

1. Tax on earnings ...................................................................... income tax

2. Tax on food, clothing. ............................................................... sales tax

3. Tax taken out of salary ........................................................ withholding tax

4. Tax on gasoline ......................................................................... gas tax

5. Tax paid on farm or home ...................................................... real estate tax

6. Tax paid on receipt of a large estate ........................................ inheritance tax

7. Tax on large amounts given a person ............................................. gift tax

8. Tax some cities charge on cars ................................................... wheel tax

9. Tax on alcohol ...................................................................... liquor tax

10. Tax on jewelry ...................................................................... luxury tax

11. Tax on profits on investments .............................................. capitol gain tax

12. Tax on gas, water, lights ......................................................... utility tax

13. Things not taxed .................................................................. tax exempt

14. Tax filing date ..................................................................... April 15th

15. Forecasting what your taxes will be ........................................... estimated tax

16. How often are estimated taxes paid .............................................. quarterly

17. Charges for parking .............................................................. parking fees

18. Charges on highways and bridges .................................................. toll tax

19. Costs added for late payment of taxes ....................................... penalty or fine

20. Taxes not paid on time ...................................................... past due - delinquent

21. A contract is an ..................................................... agreement between people

22. Anything put up to secure a loan ................................................ collateral

23. Owner of rental property ........................................................... landlord

24. Renter of property .................................................................... tenant

25. Money paid to live in someone's house ................................................ rent

26. Agreement between owner and renter ................................................. lease

27.   Papers showing ownership and title ...................................................................... deed

28.   Papers showing location, description, history of property ............................... abstract

29.   Money loaned to purchase property ............................................................... mortgage

30.   Money charged for the use of money ............................................................... interest

31.   A financial claim fixed against property .................................................................. lien

32.   Money charged to place values on property for a loan ............................ appraisal fee

3 3.   Two main forms of farm rent ............................................... percentage or cash rent

34.   Rent for boarding a pasture ...................................................................... privilege rent

35.   A fee paid to bind a contract for a time .......................................................... retainer

36.   Tax deduction on your home ...................................................... homestead exemption

# CAR & TRUCK PARTS & NEEDS
### CREATED BY GLENN SEYMOUR

1. Something worn on the head _____
2. Something cows grow _____
3. An old horse _____
4. Part of a water heating furnace _____
5. A cooling device _____
6. A furnace heat control_____
7. What toothpaste comes in_____
8. Not a porch column but a _____
9. Not a ferris wheel but a _____
10. Not a stocking cap but a _____
11. There is a padlock also _____
12. A singer named Freddie _____
13. Where you put fuel _____
14. Something to make ride smoother _____
15. Numbers & letters on front & back _____
16. Not spare ribs but _____
17. No light, no horn, motor won't turn over _____
18. Helps you on icy roads _____
19. Does not have a tail but a _____
20. Does not have sled runners but has_____
21. Doesn't have running water but a _____
22. Not known to hijack but may have a_____
23. What is the luggage compartment_____
24. Not a flower bulb but a _____
25. Maybe not a bang up party but a_____
26. For the smoker _____
27. What metal was used to trim in early years_____
28. Small farm truck _____
29. Used to haul trash _____
30. Truck you can rent _____
31. Truck for cross country hauling _____
32.. Used to haul within the community _____
33. Truck with open slat siding _____
34. Used to haul gravel, grain, etc _____
35. Not a pressure gauge but a_____
36. What you use in the radiator in cold weather _____

# CAR & TRUCK PARTS & NEEDS
## CREATED BY GLENN SEYMOUR

1. Something worn on the head.................................................................... hood
2. Something cows grow.......................................................................... horns
3. An old horse....................................................................................plug
4. Part of a water heating furnace........................................................ radiator
5. A cooling device ...................................................................................fan
6. A furnace heat control .................................................................. thermostat
7. What toothpaste comes in..................................................................tube
8. Not a porch column but a ........................................................ steering column
9. Not a ferris wheel but a............................................................ steering wheel
10. Not a stocking cap but a ............................................................ radiator cap
11. There is a padlock also.................................................................. door locks
12. A singer named Freddie ..................................................................... fender
13. Where you put fuel............................................................................gas tank
14. Something to make ride smoother ................................................shock absorber
15. Numbers & letters on front & back..............................................license plates
16. Not spare ribs but .......................................................................spare tires
17. No light, no horn, motor won't turn over ......................................dead battery
18. Helps you on icy roads .................................................................snow tires
19. Does not have a tail but a ............................................................. tail pipe
20. Does not have sled runners but has .....................................................wheels
21. Doesn't have running water but a ...............................................running board
22. Not known to hijack but may have a ..............................................Car jack
23. What is the luggage compartment .................................................... Trunk
24. Not a flower bulb but a ............................................................... Light bulb
25. Maybe not a bang up party but a............................................Blow out
26. For the smoker............................................................................Ash tray
27. What metal was used to trim in early years............................................ Brass
28. Small farm truck............................................................................. Pick up
29. Used to haul trash............................................................................ Garbage truck
30. Truck you can rent ...................................................................... U-Haul
31. Truck for cross country hauling ...................................................Semi
32. Used to haul within the community...............................................Delivery truck
33. Truck with open slat siding...........................................................Livestock truck
34. Used to haul gravel, grain, etc.............................................................Dump truck
35. Not a pressure gauge but a ............................................................ Tire gauge
36. What you use in the radiator in cold weather .......................................... Antifreeze

# ALL AROUND THE HOUSE
### CREATED BY GLENN SEYMOUR

1. Where I find myself looking at me _____

2. I have such pains in my _____

3. What sweeps clean? _____

4. Not a IV but a _____

5. Not a real energetic boy but a _____

6. The Holy Book _____

7. What coffee is served on _____

8. She is a neat _____

9. In by gone days it was a kerosene _____

10. Window trim _____

11. Container for things you don't want _____

12. Never owned a motor van but had a _____

13. Don't have a fruit tree but have a _____

14. People go door to door selling _____

15. Not rugs tossed about but _____

16. He was trying to get it off his _____

17. Something to rest your tired feet on _____

18. A book of numbers _____

19. A place for needles and pins _____

20. Where I sit to write my checks _____

21. My mailing directory _____

22. Something draped on the back of a sofa _____

23. Keys that won't fit any lock _____

24. Insures delivery of a letter _____

25. Not a Japanese cabinet but a _____

# ALL AROUND THE HOUSE
## CREATED BY GLENN SEYMOUR

1. Where I find myself looking at me.................................................... mirror

2. I have such pains in my ................................................................. chest

3. What sweeps clean?...................................................................... broom

4. Not a IV but a .....................................................................................tv

5. Not a real energetic boy but a .................................................lazy boy

6. The Holy Book................................................................................ Bible

7. What coffee is served on................................................... coffee table

8. She is a neat .................................................................................dresser

9. In by gone days it was a kerosene................................................. lamp

10. Window trim ................................................................................ drapes

11. Container for things you don't want.............................. waist basket

12. Never owned a motor van but had a............................................ divan

13. Don't have a fruit tree but have a.............................................hall tree

14. People go door to door selling.............................................magazines

15. Not rugs tossed about but .....................................................throw rugs

16. He was trying to get it off his .....................................................chest

17. Something to rest your tired feet on ......................................footstool

18. A book of numbers ....................................... telephone directory

19. A place for needles and pins ............................................ pin cushion

20. Where I sit to write my checks .......................................................desk

21. My mailing directory ..............................................address book

22. Something draped on the back of a sofa ................................... afghan

23. Keys that won't fit any lock............................................... piano

24. Insures delivery of a letter ............................................. stamp

25. Not a Japanese cabinet but a ............................................China cabinet

# THE KITCHEN
## CREATED BY GLENN SEYMOUR

1.  Where does the batter stand?.......................................................................................

2.  If it won't float it will .............................................................................................

3.  I bought a TV satellite ............................................................................................

4.  It's fun to go to the gym & watch the .....................................................................

5.  While traveling we came to a ...................................................................................

6.  The room was hot as an ...........................................................................................

7.  Why not have .............................................................................................of tea

8.  That bucket leaks like a ..........................................................................................

9.  He could not win so he threw in the..........................................................................

10. He keeps his medicine in the medicine .....................................................................

11. The young couple love to sit in the moonlight and....................................................

12. Jack Sprat and his wife licked the ........................................................... clean

13. She likes to fry in her ...............................................................................................

14. She hit him over the head with her ..........................................................................

15. To can tomatoes you must have ...............................................................................

16. That old Gentlemen is an old.....................................................................................

17. The man who throws the ball is the ..........................................................................

18. Another name for a UFO ..........................................................................................

19. Not a sandbox but a ..................................................................................................

20. Not the Rose Bowl but a ...........................................................................................

21. Not a bed sheet but a.................................................................................................

22. Not a door opener but a ............................................................................................

23. I bought a drop cloth but a........................................................................................

24. Something to brown bread.........................................................................................

25. What will take food scraps ........................................................................................

26. What tells you when it is mealtime...........................................................................

27. To make French fries you need a..............................................................................

28. What is marked ¼, ½ and 1 .....................................................................................

29. A 3 pound chicken is called a ...................................................................................

# THE KITCHEN
## CREATED BY GLENN SEYMOUR

1.  Where does the batter stand?....................................................home plate

2.  If it won't float it will ...........................................................................sink

3.  I bought a TV satellite ......................................................................dish

4.  It's fun to go to the gym & watch the...........................................tumblers

5.  While traveling we came to a ..............................................................fork

6.  The room was hot as an ....................................................................oven

7.  Why not have a ..................................................................cup of tea

8.  That bucket leaks like a.....................................................................sieve

9.  He could not win so he threw in the...............................................towel

10. He keeps his medicine in the medicine............................... cabinet

11. The young couple love to sit in the moonlight and............................ spoon

12. Jack Sprat and his wife licked the .....................................platter clean

13. She likes to fry in her .......................................................skillet

14. She hit him over the head with her ...............................rolling pin

15. To can tomatoes you must have ............................................jars

16. That old Gentlemen is an old............................................. timer

17. The man who throws the ball is the ..............................pitcher

18. Another name for a UFO ...........................................flying saucer

19. Not a sandbox but a ..................................................bread box

20. Not the Rose Bowl but a ....................................... sugar bowl

21. Not a bed sheet but a............................................. cookie sheet

22. Not a door opener but a ...........................................can opener

23. I bought a drop cloth but a.......................................dish cloth

24. Something to brown bread................................................ toaster

25. What will take food scraps............................... garbage disposal

26. What tells you when it is mealtime........................................clock

27. To make French fries you need a................................ deep fryer

28. What is marked ¼, ½ and 1 ....................................measuring cup

29. A 3 pound chicken is called a ...................................fryer  broiler

# THE HUMAN BODY
## BODY CREATED BY GLENN SEYMOUR

1.  What is an auricle ................................................................................................

2.  What is a part of a needle ...................................................................................

3.  What is a young cow ............................................................................................

4.  What is called a piggy .........................................................................................

5.  Not a high brow or low brow but an .................................................................

6.  Not a knife blade but a .......................................................................................

7.  What is the snout .................................................................................................

8.  Where is the arch .................................................................................................

9.  What is part of a corn stalk ................................................................................

10. What is a part of a tree .......................................................................................

11. If someone mistreats you, turn the other .........................................................

12. A part of a river is the .........................................................................................

13. He does not have a ...............................................................................................

14. Two parts of the bed that are parts of the body ...............................................

15. What part of a clock tells the time ....................................................................

16. What is part of a comb ........................................................................................

17. Where do you wear a watch ................................................................................

18. It makes me weak in the .....................................................................................

19. The name of a tree is ...........................................................................................

20. You get pneumonia in your ................................................................................

21. Where is the bridge .............................................................................................

# THE HUMAN BODY
## CREATED BY GLENN SEYMOUR

1.  What is an auricle................................................................................................ear

2.  What is a part of a needle.................................................................................. eye

3.  What is a young cow.........................................................................................calf

4.  What is called a piggy.......................................................................................toe

5.  Not a high brow or low brow but an............................................................. eyebrow

6.  Not a knife blade but a.................................................................... shoulder blade

7.  What is the snout.............................................................................................nose

8.  Where is the arch..............................................................................................foot

9.  What is part of a corn stalk..............................................................................ear

10. What is a part of a tree...................................................................................limb

11. If someone mistreats you, turn the other.....................................................cheek

12. A part of a river is the.................................................................................. mouth

13. He does not have a ..................................................................... leg to stand on

14. Two parts of the bed that are parts of the body...............................head - foot

15. What part of a clock tells the time ..............................................................hands

16. What is part of a comb ................................................................................. teeth

17. Where do you wear a watch......................................................................... wrist

18. It makes me weak in the ...............................................................................knees

19. The name of a tree is ...................................................................................palm

20. You get pneumonia in your............................................................................lungs

21. Where is the bridge...................................................................................... mouth

# ITEMS IN A GROCERY STORE
### WITH THE VOWELS OMITTED
### CREATED BY GLENN SEYMOUR

1.   _ l _ _   .............................................................................

2.   ch _ _ s _ ........................................................................

3.   s _ _ r cr _ _ m .............................................................

4.   _ n _ _ n d _ p ...............................................................

5.   _ r _ ng _  j _ _ c _ ........................................................

6.   s _ l _ d  dr _ ss _ ng ...................................................

7.   t _ m _ t _  s _ _ p .........................................................

8.   p _ _ n _ t  b _ tt _ r .....................................................

9.   cl _ m ch _ wd _ r s _ _ p ............................................

10.  c _ c _ _   ........................................................................

11.  d _ m _ n _ s _ g _ r ......................................................

12.  _ _ d _ z _ d  s _ lt .........................................................

13.  s _ g _   .............................................................................

14.  t _ m _ r _ c   ...................................................................

15.  q _ _ k _ r  _ _ ts   .........................................................

16.  ch _ rr _ _ s   ...................................................................

17.  r _ m _ n  m _ _ l  b r _ _ d ........................................

18.  wh _ _ t _ _ s   .................................................................

19.  f _ lg _ rs  c _ ff _ _   .....................................................

20.  l _ pt _ n  t _ _   ..............................................................

21.  m _ lt _  m _ _ l   ............................................................

22.  ch _ c _ l _ t _ e  m _ lk ...............................................

23.  r _ _ s _ n  br _ n   ..........................................................

24.  st _ r  k _ st  t _ n _   ......................................................

25.  s _ lm _ n   ........................................................................

26.  c _ d _ r   ..........................................................................

# ITEMS IN A GROCERY STORE
## WITH THE VOWELS OMITTED
### CREATED BY GLENN SEYMOUR

27. dr _ _ d  _ pr _ c _ ts .................................................................................

28. c _ d  l _ v _ r  _ _ l ...............................................................................

29. cr _ n _ l _  _ _ l ..................................................................................

30. s _ rd _ n _ s .........................................................................................

31. gr _ p _  fr _ _ t  j _ _ c _ ...................................................................

32. d _ c _ d  b _ _ ts .................................................................................

33. l _ m _ n  _ xtr _ ct .............................................................................

34. _ r _ _  c _ _ k _ _ s ............................................................................

35. cr _ nb _ rry  s _ _ c _ ........................................................................

36. t _ nd _ rl _ _ n ...................................................................................

37. m _ nc _  m _ _ t  p _ _ ......................................................................

38. l _ v _ r ..................................................................................................

39. p _ rk  s _ _ s _ g _ ............................................................................

40. r _ _ nd  st _ _ k ..................................................................................

41. h _ mb _ rg _ r .....................................................................................

42. sp _ c _ d  h _ m .................................................................................

43. b _ _ f  r _ _ st ....................................................................................

44. fr _ nch  _ n _ _ n  s _ _ p ................................................................

# ITEMS IN A GROCERY STORE
## WITH THE VOWELS OMITTED
### CREATED BY GLENN SEYMOUR

1.  _ l _ _ .............................................. oleo

2.  ch _ _ s _ ............................................ cheese

3.  s _ _ r cr _ _ m ................................... sour cream

4.  _ n _ _ n d _ p ..................................... onion dip

5.  _ r _ ng _ j _ _ c _ ............................... orange juice

6.  s _ l _ d dr _ ss _ ng ........................ salad dressing

7.  t _ m _ t _ s _ _ p ............................... tomato soup

8.  p _ _ n _ t b _ tt _ r ........................... peanut butter

9.  cl _ m ch _ wd _ r s _ _ p ................. clam chowder soup

10. c _ c _ _ .............................................. cocoa

11. d _ m _ n _ s _ g _ r ......................... domino sugar

12. _ _ d _ z _ d s _ lt ............................. iodized salt

13. s _ g _ .............................................. sage

14. t _ m _ r _ c ...................................... tumeric

15. q _ _ k _ r _ _ ts .............................. quaker oats

16. ch _ rr _ _ s ...................................... cherries

17. r _ m _ n m _ _ l b r _ _ d ............. roman meal bread

18. wh _ _ t _ _ s ................................... wheaties

19. f _ lg _ rs c _ ff _ _ ....................... folgers coffee

20. l _ pt _ n t _ _ ................................. lipton tea

21. m _ lt m _ _ l .................................. malto meal

22. ch _ c _ l _ t _ e m _ lk ................. chocolate milk

23. r _ _ s _ n br _ n ........................... raisin bran

24. st _ r k _ st t _ n _ ...................... star kist tuna

25. s _ lm _ n .......................................... salmon

26. c _ d _ r ............................................. cider

# ITEMS IN A GROCERY STORE
## WITH THE VOWELS OMITTED
### CREATED BY GLENN SEYMOUR

27.  dr _ _ d  _ pr _ c _ ts ......................... dried apricots

28.  c _ d  l _ v _ r  _ _ l ......................... cod liver oil

29.  cr _ n _ l _  _ _ l ............................. cranola oil

30.  s _ rd _ n _ s ................................... sardines

31.  gr _ p _  fr _ _ t  j _ _ c _ ................ grapefruit juice

32.  d _ c _ d  b _ _ ts ............................ diced beets

33.  l _ m _ n  _ xtr _ ct ........................ lemon extract

34.  _ r _ _  c _ _ k _ _ s ........................ oreo cookies

35.  cr _ nb _ rry  s _ _ c _ .................... cranberry sauce

36.  t _ nd _ rl _ _ n ................................ tenderloin

37.  m _ nc _  m _ _ t  p _ _ ................ mince meat pie

38.  l _ v _ r ........................................... liver

39.  p _ rk  s _ _ s _ g _ ......................... pork sausage

40.  r _ _ nd  st _ _ k .............................. round steak

41.  h _ mb _ rg _ r ................................. hamburger

42.  sp _ c _ d  h _ m ............................. spiced ham

43.  b _ _ f  r _ _ st ................................ beef roast

44.  fr _ nch  _ n _ _ n  s _ _ p ............ french onion soup

# DEFINITIONS

# DEFINITIONS
CREATED BY GLENN SEYMOUR

1. Gambling City_____

2. Rock from volcano _____

3. Genuine_____

4. Picnic pests _____

5. Wee small drink _____

6. Window glass _____

7. Winter toy _____

8. Mistake _____

9. Beer glass_____

10. Treaty _____

11. Back talk _____

12. Veranda _____

13. Strew _____

14. Flexible _____

15. Foundation _____

16. Conceal _____

17. Ignite _____

18. Bird's home _____

19. Cobra_____

20. Single man_____

21. Clue _____

22. Startle _____

23. Eyesore _____

24 Finishes _____

25. Ancient _____

26. Steep rock _____

27. G. I. _____

28. Famous garden _____

29. Loan _____

30. Site_____

31. Ships record_____

32. Human _____

33. Rodent_____

34. Indian tent_____

35. Assistant _____

36. Two words in a wedding _____

37. Journey _____

38. S. O. S. _____

39. Blue gill _____

40. First man _____

41. First Woman _____

42. Competent _____

43. Ice cream holder _____

44. Fruit pastry _____

45. Sibling _____

46. Healthy _____

47. Eerie _____

48. Residence _____

49. Onset_____

50. Auctioneer last word _____

# DEFINITIONS
CREATED BY GLENN SEYMOUR

1. Gambling City.................. Las Vegas
2. Rock from volcano ..................... lava
3. Genuine ...........................real
4. Picnic pests....................................ants
5. Wee small drink........................ sip
6. Window glass............................pane
7. Winter toy ..................................... sled
8. Mistake ........................................ error
9. Beer glass ..............................stein
10. Treaty ......................................pact
11. Back talk ..............................sass
12. Veranda....................................porch
13. Strew.......................................scatter
14. Flexible....................................elastic
15. Foundation .........................base
16. Conceal....................................hide
17. Ignite ............................... light
18. Bird's home..............................nest
19. Cobra.......................... snake
20. Single man..........................bachelor
21. Clue ......................................hint
22. Startle ................................. scare
23. Eyesore ............................... sty
24. Finishes....................................ends
25. Ancient...............................old
26. Steep rock ........................ cliff
27. G. I. ................................. soldier
28. Famous garden .........................Eden
29. Loan..........................grant use of
30. Site..............................................spot
31. Ships record..........................log
32. Human...................................person
33. Rodent...................................rat
34. Indian tent............................teepee
35. Assistant................................ aide
36. Two words in a wedding ...........I do
37. Journey...................................trip
38. S. O. S.........................distress signal
39. Blue gill ................................fish
40. First man ............................. Adam
41. First Woman............................ Eve
42. Competent...................................able
43. Ice cream holder ...................... cone
44. Fruit pastry....................................pie
45. Sibling ...............................child
46. Healthy ........................................ well
47. Eerie.................................... odd
48. Residence................................. home
49. Onset ...................................starts
50. Auctioneer last word...................sold

# DEFINITIONS
## CREATED BY GLENN SEYMOUR

1. Teachers favorite _____
2. Headman _____
3. Entire _____
4. Feel sick _____
5. Auction _____
6. Wedding band _____
7. Accomplish _____
8. Dine _____
9. Aware of _____
10. Ice pellets _____
11. Ship of the desert _____
12. Big white bear _____
13. Encounter _____
14. Chopping tool _____
15. Hospital worker _____
16. Lending a hand _____
17. Midday _____
18. Hospital division _____
19. Coins _____
20. Guide _____
21. Ache _____
22. Listen _____
23. Lease _____
24. Ere _____
25. Quarry _____
26. Peril _____
27. Flame _____
28. Sun _____
29. Young boy _____
30. Press _____
31. Egg drink _____
32. Small _____
33. Spelling contest _____
34. Albatross _____
35. Large _____
36. Rip _____
37. Alphabet _____
38. Church seat _____
39. Swap _____
40. Attempt _____
41. Create _____
42. Rumba _____
43. Foreman _____
44. Mix _____
45. Respond _____
46. Once around the track _____
47. Mother or Father _____
48. Two letters before noon _____
49. Band leader _____
50. Two letters after noon _____

# DEFINITIONS
## CREATED BY GLENN SEYMOUR

| | | |
|---|---|---|
| 1. | Teachers favorite......................pet | |
| 3. | Entire....................................... all | |
| 5. | Auction ...................................sale | |
| 7. | Accomplish.............................do | |
| 9. | Aware of.................................know | |
| 11. | Ship of the desert...................camel | |
| 13. | Encounter .............................meet | |
| 15. | Hospital worker .....................nurse | |
| 17. | Midday................................... noon | |
| 19. | Coins ..................................... money | |
| 21. | Ache .......................................pain | |
| 23. | Lease....................................... rent | |
| 25. | Quarry ...................... stone mine | |
| 27. | Flame.......................................fire | |
| 29. | Young boy...............................lad | |
| 31. | Egg drink................................eggnog | |
| 33. | Spelling contest....................... bee | |
| 35. | Large.......................................huge | |
| 37. | Alphabet .................................letters | |
| 39. | Swap ...................................... trade | |
| 41. | Create .....................................make | |
| 43. | Foreman...................................boss | |
| 45. | Respond ................................. answer | |
| 47. | Mother or Father ................. parent | |
| 49. | Band leader ................. conductor | |

| | | |
|---|---|---|
| 2. | Headsman ............................... boss |
| 4. | Feel sick ..................................ail |
| 6. | Wedding band ..........................ring |
| 8. | Dine.........................................eat |
| 10. | Ice pellets................................ sleet |
| 12. | Big white bear ..........................polar |
| 14. | Chopping tool............................ ax |
| 16. | Lending a hand.........................help |
| 18. | Hospital division ..................... ward |
| 20. | Guide ..................................... leader |
| 22. | Listen .....................................heed |
| 24. | Ere ......................................... before |
| 26. | Peril........................................danger |
| 28. | Sun ........................................ sol |
| 30. | Press ......................................iron |
| 32. | Small ...............................tiny- wee |
| 34. | Albatross..................................bird |
| 36. | Rip .......................................... tear |
| 38. | Church seat ..............................pew |
| 40. | Attempt........................................try |
| 42. | Rumba ....................................dance |
| 44. | Mix..........................................stir |
| 46. | Once around the track................lap |
| 48. | Two letters before noon..............am |
| 50. | Two letters after noon................pm |

# DEFINITIONS
CREATED BY GLENN SEYMOUR

1. Small body of water _____
2. Huge dry land _____
3. Quill _____
4. Clinched hand _____
5. Earth tremor _____
6. Cut_____
7. Energy _____
8. Dawn_____
9. Kin_____
10. Jump _____
11. Nightbird_____
12. Orient _____
13. Sixth sense_____
14. Bottomless_____
15. Ajar _____
16. Dusk _____
17. Underground drain _____
18. Bind_____
19. Unreal _____
20. Never ending_____
21. Pocketbook _____
22. Orange rind_____
23. Unruly crowd _____
24. Torment_____
25. Gambling cubes_____
26. Endure_____
27. Groan _____
28. Fetch _____
29. Hermit_____
30. Break suddenly _____
31. Sparkle_____
32. Party giver _____
33. Commence _____
34. Evil _____
35. Ledge_____
36. Prior _____
37. Garret _____
38. Omit _____
39. Animal coat_____
40. Tress _____
41. Vanish _____
42. Sample food_____
43. Frost a cake _____
44. Brain storm _____
45. Cushion_____
46. Money till _____
47. Doctor visitor _____
48. Detest _____
49. Jumble _____
50. Winter flakes _____

# DEFINITIONS
## CREATED BY GLENN SEYMOUR

1. Small body of water.............. puddle
2. Huge dry land.........................desert
3. Quill ....................................pen
4. Clinched hand .............................. fist
5. Earth tremor ......................quake
6. Cut.................................slice - chop
7. Energy...............................pep
8. Dawn.....................early morning
9. Kin ..................................relative
10. Jump.....................................leap
11. Night bird ...........................owl
12. Orient....................................east
13. Sixth sense .........................csp
14. Bottomless............................pit
15. Ajar ....................................open
16. Dusk ................................evening
17. Underground drain ......sewer – tile
18. Bind.........................................tie
19. Unreal ...............................fake
20. Never ending ..........................ever
21. Pocketbook.........................purse
22. Orange rind............................. peel
23. Unruly crowd ........................ mob
24. Torment.................................tease
25. Gambling cubes......................dice
26. Endure ................................. last
27. Groan ............................... moan
28. Fetch.................................bring
29. Hermit.............................. loaner
30. Break suddenly ...................... snap
31. Sparkle .......................glow- shine
32. Party giver ............................host
33. Commence.................begin - start
34. Evil ........................................bad
35. Ledge............................... shelf
36. Prior ........................................ before
37. Garret...............................attic
38. Omit...................................leave out
39. Animal coat............................pelt
40. Tress ........................lock of hair
41. Vanish ........................ disappear
42. Sample food ............................ taste
43. Frost a cake................................ ice
44. Brain storm ...........................idea
45. Cushion.................................Pad
46. Money till. ...................Cash register
47. Doctor visitor...................... patient
48. Detest ...........................................hate
49. Jumble ...........................mess
50. Winter flakes.......................... snow

56

# DEFINITIONS
CREATED BY GLENN SEYMOUR

1.  Affirmative _____
2.  Out of order _____
3.  Depart _____
4.  Miserly _____
5.  About _____
6.  Pan cover _____
7.  Oodles _____
8.  Forty winks _____
9.  Secondhand _____
10. Garb _____
11. Nod _____
12. Propose _____
13. Small parcel of land _____
14. Spin _____
15. Mimic _____
16. Stow _____
17. Lead role _____
18. Lubricate _____
19. Storm center _____
20. Verse _____
21. Glance _____
22. Prohibit _____
23. Price _____
24. Seek _____
25. Worth _____
26. Auction offer _____
27. Flower support _____
28. Oil boat _____
29. Hairpiece _____
30. Tow _____
31. Outcome _____
32. Saturate _____
33. Sound _____
34. Slumber _____
35. Railroad depot _____
36. Cigar residue _____
37. Storage room for clothes _____
38. Whopper _____
39. Bottle stopper _____
40. Baby Bed _____
41. Paid player _____
42. Teenager _____
43. Winter storm _____
44. Misplace _____
45. Not at home _____
46. High card _____
47. Cozy room _____
48. Afternoon social _____
49. Noxious plant _____
50. Woe is me _____

# DEFINITIONS
## CREATED BY GLENN SEYMOUR

1.  Affirmative ................................ yes
2.  Out of order ........................... broken
3.  Depart ................................. leave
4.  Miserly ................................ stingy
5.  About ................................. almost
6.  Pan cover ................................ lid
7.  Oodles ................................. lots
8.  Forty winks ............................... nap
9.  Secondhand ........................... used
10. Garb ............................. clothing
11. Nod .......................... bob your head
12. Propose ............................. suggest
13. Small parcel of land ................. acre
14. Spin ................................... twirl
15. Mimic ................................. copy
16. Stow ...................... hide away
17. Lead role ............................. star
18. Lubricate ................................. oil
19. Storm center ....................... eye
20. Verse .............................. poem
21. Glance .......................... look - peek
22. Prohibit ................................ ban
23. Price .......................... cost - fee
24. Seek ....................... search - hunt
25. Worth .............................. value
26. Auction offer ............................. bid
27. Flower support ....................... stem
28. Oil boat ............................ tanker
29. Hairpiece .................. wig- toupee
30. Tow .......................... pull - drag
31. Outcome ........................... result
32. Saturate ............................. soak
33. Sound ........................... noise
34. Slumber .............................. sleep
35. Railroad depot ................. station
36. Cigar residue ............................. ash
37. Storage room for clothes ....... closet
38. Whopper ............................... fib
39. Bottle stopper ........ cork - cap - lid
40. Baby bed ............................. crib
41. Paid player ......................... pro
42. Teenager ........................... adolescent
43. Winter storm ................... blizzard
44. Misplace ............................ lose
45. Not at home .......................... away
46. High card ............................ ace
47. Cozy room ........................ den
48. Afternoon social ...................... tea
49. Noxious plant ................... weed
50. Woe is me ........................... alas

# DEFINITIONS
CREATED BY GLENN SEYMOUR

1. Illuminated _____
2. Leave out _____
3. Cobra _____
4. Newsboy cry _____
5. Single man _____
6. Shoestring _____
7. Clue _____
8. Startle _____
9. Steep rock _____
10. G. I. _____
11. Ancient _____
12. Famous garden _____
13. Heap _____
14. Ship's record _____
15. Rodent _____
16. Human _____
17. Best friend _____
18. Purchase _____
19. Site _____
20. Assistant _____
21. Birds home _____
22. Wigwam _____
23. Journey _____
24. S. 0. S. _____
25. Blue gill _____
26. Woody plant _____
27. Sheriff's group _____
28. Wound remains _____
29. Soft drink _____
30. That thing _____
31. Baby's napkin _____
32. Eskimo's home _____
33. Give off light _____
34. Walk in water _____
35. Take to court _____
36. Cut grain _____
37. Breathe hard _____
38. First gardener _____
39. Prayer ending _____
40. Not as many _____
41. Armed conflict _____
42. Undo a knot _____
43. Butter substitute _____
44. Wear away _____
45. Weighing device _____
46. Walk in water _____
47. Bullring cheer _____
48. Pa's mate _____
49. College official _____
50. Make lace _____

# DEFINITIONS
### CREATED BY GLENN SEYMOUR

1. Illuminated ................................lit
2. Leave out ................................. omit
3. Cobra ........................... snake
4. Newsboy cry ...........................extra
5. Single man.................... bachelor
6. Shoestring ..................................lace
7. Clue ....................................hint
8. Startle.................................scare
9. Steep rock ...........................cliff
10. G. I. ..................................soldier
11. Ancient ..............................old
12. Famous garden ...................... Eden
13. Heap ...................................pile
14. Ship's record ..........................log
15. Rodent........................... rat- mouse
16. Human.................................. person
17. Best friend ..............................pal
18. Purchase .................................buy
19. Site .....................................spot
20. Assistant ................................ aid
21. Birds home ........................ nest
22. Wigwam ...................... Indian tent
23. Journey................................trip
24. S.O. S. ..................................help
25. Blue gill ..............................fish
26. Woody plant..............................tree
27. Sheriffs group.........................posse
28. Wound remains........................ scar
29. Soft drink............................ soda
30. That thing........................................it
31. Baby's napkin ...........................bib
32. Eskimo's home ..........................igloo
33. Give off light............................shine
34. Walk in water............................ wade
35. Take to court ...........................sue
36. Cut grain................................harvest
37. Breathe hard............................pant
38. First gardener..........................Adam
39. Prayer ending........................amen
40. Not as many ............................. less
41. Armed conflict....................war
42. Undo a knot ............................ untie
43. Butter substitute ....................Oleo
44. Wear away .................................erode
45. Weighing device ....................scale
46. Walk in water............................ wade
47. Bullring cheer ........................ole
48. Pa's mate .................................Ma
49. College official ......................dean
50. Make lace................................tat

# DEFINITIONS
CREATED BY GLENN SEYMOUR

1.  Crucifix _____
2.  Citrus _____
3.  Crumb _____
4.  Scar _____
5.  Policeman _____
6.  String _____
7.  Border _____
8.  Alit _____
9.  Couple _____
10. Elevate _____
11. Boast _____
12. Excavate _____
13. Fix _____
14. Far _____
15. Cloth _____
16. Free _____
17. Stitch _____
18. Applaud _____
19. Slant _____
20. Temporary bed _____
21. Dentures _____
22. Veranda _____
23. Creep _____
24. Title _____
25. Faucet _____
26. Seabird _____
27. Train Tracks _____
28. Migraine _____
29. Arid _____
30. Tepid _____
31. Hog fat _____
32. Beef fat _____
33. Wren _____
34. Moist _____
35. Rollaway _____
36. Desist _____
37. Detour _____
38. Demolish _____
39. Come infirst _____
40. Support _____
41. Fracture _____
42. Dusk _____
43. Sign showing way out _____
44. Ajar _____
45. Bottomless _____
46. Sixth sense _____
47. Bind _____
48. Orient _____
49. Night bird _____
50. Jump _____

# DEFINITIONS
CREATED BY GLENN SEYMOUR

1. Crucifix .................................cross
2. Citrus .................................fruit
3. Crumb................................ morsel
4. Scar.................................cut mark
5. Policeman .................................cop
6. String.................................cord
7. Border .................................edge
8. Alit.................................landed
9. Couple......................... two people
10. Elevate.................................rate
11. Boast.................................brag
12. Excavate.................................dig
13. Fix ..................... repair - mend
14. Far ..................... distant
15. Cloth ..................... fabric
16. Free.................................rid of
17. Stitch ..................... sews
18. Applaud ..................... clap
19. Slant..................... slope
20. Temporary bed ..................... cot
21. Dentures .................................teeth
22. Veranda ..................... porch
23. Creep.................................crawl
24. Title.................................name
25. Faucet.................................tap
26. Seabird.................................gull
27. Train Tracks .........................rails
28. Migraine......................... headache
29. Arid ..................... dry
30. Tepid ..................... warm
31. Hog fat .........................lard
32. Beef fat.................................tallow
33. Wren.................................bird
34. Moist.................................damp-wet
35. Rollaway .........................bed
36. Desist ..................... stop
37. Detour...............go around bypass
38. Demolish ..................... destroy
39. Come in first ..................... win
40. Support..................... rafter
41. Fracture.........................break
42. Dusk.................................evening
43. Sign showing way out ...............exit
44. Ajar.................................open
45. Bottomless.........................pit
46. Sixth sense.................................esp
47. Bind.........................tie
48. Orient.................................east
49. Night bird .........................owl
50. Jump.................................leap

# DEFINITIONS
## CREATED BY GLENN SEYMOUR

1. Pile up _____
2. Stitch _____
3. Noisy _____
4. Tiny _____
5. Healthy _____
6. Away _____
7. Area _____
8. Angry _____
9. Difficult _____
10. Hay field _____
11. Unruly crowd _____
12. Help _____
13. Thaw _____
14. Dine _____
15. Lettuce dish _____
16. Caution _____
17. Entire _____
18. Egg Drink _____
19. Winter toy _____
20. Writing fluid _____
21. Adhesive _____
22. At home _____
23. Labor _____
24. Young boy _____
25. Slippery fish _____
26. Close by _____
27. At no time _____
28. Comes in first _____
29. Frozen water _____
30. Rowing device _____
31. The center _____
32. Not allowed _____
33. Picnic pest _____
34. Sturdy tree _____
35. Practice boxing _____
36. Busy insect _____
37. Poke fun _____
38. Jean material _____
39. Legal title _____
40. Leave out _____
41. Best friend _____
42. Pod vegetable _____
43. Title of respect _____
44. Small drink _____
45. Wedding words _____
46. Even score _____
47. Map book _____
48. High card _____
49. Raw material _____
50. Chicago lake _____

# DEFINITIONS
## CREATED BY GLENN SEYMOUR

1. Pile up .................................. stack
2. Stitch ........................................ sew
3. Noisy ..................................... loud
4. Tiny ............................... wee- small
5. Healthy ............................... well
6. Away ..................................... gone
7. Area ...................................... space
8. Angry ..................................... mad
9. Difficult .............................. hard
10. Hay field ........................... meadow
11. Unruly crowd ....................... mob
12. Help ........................... assist- aid
13. Thaw .................................... melt
14. Dine ........................................ eat
15. Lettuce dish ........................ salad
16. Caution ............................... warn
17. Entire ....................................... all
18. Egg Drink ......................... eggnog
19. Winter toy ............................ sled
20. Writing fluid ........................ ink
21. Adhesive ............................ paste
22. At home .................................. Ill
23. Labor .................................... work
24. Young boy .............................. lad
25. Slippery fish .......................... eel
26. Close by ............................... near
27. At no time ........................... never
28. Comes in first .................. winner
29. Frozen water .......................... ice
30. Rowing device ....................... oar
31. The center ........................... core
32. Not allowed ...................... forbid
33. Picnic pest ............................ ant
34. Sturdy tree .............................. oak
35. Practice boxing .................... spar
36. Busy insect ............................ bee
37. Poke fun ............................. tease
38. Jean material ..................... denim
39. Legal title ........................... deed
40. Leave out ............................ omit
41. Best friend ............................ pal
42. Pod vegetable ....................... pea
43. Title of respect ...................... sir
44. Small drink ............................ sip
45. Wedding words .................... I do
46. Even score ............................. tie
47. Map book ........................... atlas
48. High card ............................... ace
49. Raw material ......................... ore
50. Chicago lake .................. Michigan

# DEFINITIONS
## CREATED BY GLENN SEYMOUR

1. Bottle stopper _____
2. Baby Bed _____
3. Teenager _____
4. Paid Player _____
5. Winter storm _____
6. Not at home _____
7. Misplace _____
8. Afternoon Social _____
9. High Card _____
10. Cozy Room _____
11. Noxious plant _____
12. Church Bench _____
13. College Official _____
14. Take To Court _____
15. Make Lace _____
16. Cut Grain _____
17. Bus Station _____
18. Breathe hard _____
19. Sheriffs group _____
20. Roof edge _____
21. Wound remains _____
22. First Gardner _____
23. Second Hand _____
24. Birds Home _____
25. Diamond Weight _____
26. Prayer Ending _____
27. Summer Drink _____
28. Not As Many _____
29. Not As Many _____
30. That Thing _____
31. Armed Conflict _____
32. Caustic Substance _____
33. Undo a knot _____
34. Soft Drink _____
35. Butter Substitute _____
36. Pancake Topping _____
37. Ma's Mate _____
38. Shopping Center _____
39. Wear Away _____
40. Baby's Napkin _____
41. Weighing Device _____
42. In This Place _____
43. Newsboy's shout _____
44. Indian Home _____
45. Line of Mountains _____
46. Woody Plant _____
47. Give Off Light _____
48. Bullring Cheer _____
49. Walk in Water _____
50. Eskimo's Home _____

# DEFINITIONS
## CREATED BY GLENN SEYMOUR

1. Bottle stopper ................ cork - cap
2. Baby Bed........................... crib
3. Teenager.......................... adolescent
4. Paid Player.................................pro
5. Winter storm.....................blizzard
6. Not at home ............................ out
7. Misplace.............................lose
8. Afternoon Social .........................tea
9. High Card..............................ace
10. Cozy Room .............................. den
11. Noxious plant.....................weed
12. Church Bench.........................pew
13. College Official ..................... dean
14. Take To Court .......................... sue
15. Make Lace...................tat - crochet
16. Cut Grain ............................ harvest
17. Bus Station..............depot terminal
18. Breathe hard........................... pant
19. Sheriffs group .......................... posse
20. Roof edge................................ eave
21. Wound remains ............scar - scab
22. First Gardner ......................... Adam
23. Second Hand............................used
24. Birds Home ................................nest
25. Diamond Weight .................... carat
26. Prayer Ending.......................... Amen
27. Summer Drink...........Lemon Aide
28. Not As Many.............................less
29. Not As Many ......................... fewer
30. That Thing.................................it
31. Armed Conflict.......................... war
32. Caustic Substance........................lye
33. Undo A Knot...........................untie
34. Soft Drink.................................soda
35. Butter Substitute ...................... oleo
36. Pancake Topping .................... syrup
37. Ma's Mate..................................... Pa
38. Shopping Center....................... mall
39. Wear Away.............................erode
40. Baby's Napkin ............................bib
41. Weighing Device ..................... scale
42. In This Place........................... here
43. Newsboy's shout ......................extra
44. Indian Home...........................tepee
45. Line of Mountains ................. range
46. Woody Plant ........................... tree
47. Give Off Light ............ shine - glow
48. Bullring Cheer ........................Ole
49. Walk in Water .......................wade
50. Eskimo's home ........................ igloo

# FLOWERS & TREES

# NAMES OF FLOWERS IN SONGS
## CREATED BY GLENN SEYMOUR

1.   Mexicali _____

2.   When you wore a _____ and I wore a big _____

3.   The _____ Of Texas

4.   My Wild Irish _____

5.   Tiptoe through the _____

6.   Underneath _____

7.   Ramblin _____

8.   Honey Suckle _____

9.   _____ Blossom Time

10.  Lonely Little _____ in an onion patch

# NAMES OF FLOWERS IN SONGS
CREATED BY GLENN SEYMOUR

1.  Mexicali ................................................................................................ Rose

2.  When you wore a........ Tulip............and I wore a big ..................................... Red Rose

3.  The................................................Yellow Rose ............................................. Of Texas

4.  My Wild Irish.......................................................................................... Rose

5.  Tiptoe through the ........................................................................................Tulips

6.  Underneath ................................................................................... The Mistletoe

7.  Rambling ..............................................................................................Rose

8.  Honey Suckle ........................................................................................ Rose

9.  Apple ............................................................................................ Blossom Time

10. Lonely Little ...................................Petunia .......................................in an onion patch

# WHAT TREE IS THIS?

## CREATED BY GLENN SEYMOUR

1. What some children call their Grandpa _____
2. A tree that cries _____
3. The old oaken bucket _____
4. A tree that blooms in the early spring _____
5. Part of a glove _____
6. Wood used to make a hope chest _____
7. A stole _____
8. A syrup made from _____
9. Whiskers like fuzz on a _____
10. Not silk wood but _____
11. A slippery tree _____
12. Tree that loses its leaves in spring _____
13. Shoes come in _____
14. Not a sourball tree but a _____
15. If eaten green it puckers your mouth _____
16. Color of a rosebud _____
17. Not a cat wood but a _____
18. Another word for black _____
19. What the village smithy stood under _____
20. A young man gets all dressed up _____
21. Very soft wood _____
22. President Johnson's first name _____
23. What is used as a farm fence _____
24. What tree is shell bark _____
25. Not me but _____
26. Sounds like a sneeze _____
27. What did Jack Homer pull out of a pie _____
28. You can sit under this with nobody but me _____
29. This tree bears long beans _____
30. What is left after a cigar is smoked _____

# WHAT TREE IS THIS?
## CREATED BY GLENN SEYMOUR

1. What some children call their Grandpa.................................................................pawpaw
2. A tree that cries.................................................................weeping willow
3. The old oaken bucket.................................................................oak
4. A tree that blooms in the early spring.................................................................tulip
5. Part of a glove.................................................................palm
6. Wood used to make a hope chest.................................................................cedar
7. A stole.................................................................fir
8. A syrup make from.................................................................maple
9. Whiskers like fuzz on a.................................................................peach
10. Not silkwood but.................................................................cottonwood
11. A slippery tree.................................................................slippery elm
12. Tree that loses its leaves in spring.................................................................pin oak
13. Shoes come in pairs.................................................................pear
14. Not a sourball tree but a.................................................................lemon tree
15. If eaten green it puckers your mouth.................................................................persimmon
16. Color of a rosebud.................................................................red bud
17. Not a catwood tree but a.................................................................dogwood
18. Another word for black.................................................................ebony tree
19. What the village smithy stood under.................................................................chestnut
20. A young man gets all dressed up.................................................................spruce
21. Very soft wood.................................................................balsam
22. President Johnson's first name.................................................................Linden
23. What is used as a farm fence.................................................................hedge
24. What tree is shell bark.................................................................hickory
25. Not me but.................................................................yew
26. Sounds like a sneeze.................................................................cashew
27. What did Jack Homer pull out of a pie.................................................................plum
28. You can sit under this with nobody but me.................................................................apple
29. This tree bears long beans.................................................................catalpa
30. What is left after a cigar is smoked.................................................................ash

# PARTS OF A TREE
CREATED BY GLENN SEYMOUR

1. A page in a book is also called _____

2. An arm or leg is called _____

3. Small piece of a limb is called _____

4. A piece of silverware is called _____

5. What a dog does _____

6. What we store things in _____

7. Foundation of a tree is _____

8. Sometimes thread gets into a _____

# PARTS OF A TREE
## CREATED BY GLENN SEYMOUR

1. A page in a book is also called ................................................................................. leaf

2. An arm or leg is called ........................................................................................... limb

3. Small piece of a limb is called ................................................................................ twig

4. A piece of silverware is called ................................................................................ fork

5. What a dog does ..................................................................................................... bark

6. What we store things in .......................................................................................... trunk

7. Foundation of a tree is ........................................................................................... roots

8. Sometimes thread gets into a .................................................................................. knot

# GEOGRAPHY

# ITEMS IN CONNECTION WITH STATE, COUNTRY, ETC

CREATED BY GLENN SEYMOUR

1. Cleanser _____

2. Toast _____

3. Oatmeal _____

4. Nut _____

5. Ham _____

6. Dog (Great) _____

7. Baked _____

8. Measles _____

9. Muffin _____

10. Sausage _____

11. Beef _____

12. Punch _____

13. Rice _____

14. Cheese _____

15. Steak _____

16. Fries _____

17. Onion _____

18. Potato _____

19. Thistle _____

20. Elm Tree _____

21. Hat _____

22. Waltz _____

23. Violet _____

24. Rangers _____

25. Dressing _____

26. Cream Cheese _____

27. Airline _____

28. Pony _____

29. Sweeper _____

30. Combine _____

31. Watch _____

32. Penny _____

33. Candle _____

34. Tape _____

35. Rug _____

36. Dells _____

37. Horse _____

38. Rifle _____

39. A dance _____

40. Kind of wood _____

# ITEMS IN CONNECTION WITH STATE, COUNTRY, ETC

CREATED BY GLENN SEYMOUR

1. Cleanser ...................................Dutch
2. Toast.......................................... French
3. Oatmeal .............................Quaker
4. Nut ........................................... Brazil
5. Ham............................... Virginia
6. Dog (Great) ............................. Dane
7. Baked ................................. Alaska
8. Measles ...............................German
9. Muffin .................................English
10. Sausage ....................................Polish
11. Beef.......................................Italian
12. Punch................................Hawaiian
13. Rice.............................. Spanish
14. Cheese............................ Wisconsin
15. Steak........................... Swiss
16. Fries........................................ French
17. Onion.................................Spanish
18. Potato....................................... Idaho
19. Thistle............................ Canada
20. Elm Tree .............................. Chinese
21. Hat........................................Panama
22. Waltz .................................Tennessee
23. Violet.............................. African
24. Rangers.........................................Texas
25. Dressing.................................French
26. Cream Cheese............. Philadelphia
27. Airline............................. American
28. Pony .....................Shetland Islands
29. Sweeper................................ Eureka
30. Combine............................. Holland
31. Watch .............................. Elgin
32. Penny ......................................Lincoln
33. Candle...................................Roman
34. Tape..........................................Scotch
35. Rug .....................................Persian
36. Dells ................................. Wisconsin
37. Horse................. Arabian - Belgium
38. Rifle........................................Remington
39. A dance ..........................Charleston
40. Kind of wood ................... Oakwood

# WHAT STATE IS THIS CITY IN?
## (Most of these are NOT capitals)
CREATED BY GLENN SEYMOUR

1. Nome _____

2. Little Rock _____

3. Yuma _____

4. Mobile _____

5. Denver _____

6. Hartford _____

7. Orlando _____

8. Dover _____

9. Macon _____

10. Honolulu _____

11. Boise _____

12. Evansville _____

13. Keokuk _____

14. Decatur _____

15. Wichita _____

16. Louisville _____

17. Baton Rouge _____

18. Bangor _____

19. Annapolis _____

20. Boston _____

21. Holland _____

22. St. Paul _____

23. Bullock _____

24. Butte _____

25. Branson _____

26. Lincoln _____

27. Utica _____

28. Trenton _____

29. Santa Fe _____

30. Concord _____

31. Charlotte _____

32. Bismarck _____

33. Akron _____

34. Enid _____

35. Madison _____

36. Nashville _____

37. Richmond _____

38. Charleston _____

39. C4eyenne _____

40. Tacoma _____

41. Mo11tpelier _____

42. Austin _____

# WHAT STATE IS THIS CITY IN?
## (Most of these are NOT capitals)
CREATED BY GLENN SEYMOUR

| | | | | |
|---|---|---|---|---|
| 1. | Nome......Alaska | 2. | Little Rock......Arkansas |
| 3. | Yuma......Arizona | 4. | Mobile......Alabama |
| 5. | Denver......Colorado | 6. | Hartford......Connecticut |
| 7. | Orlando......Florida | 8. | Dover....Delaware New Hampshire |
| 9. | Macon......Georgia | 10. | Honolulu......Hawaii |
| 11. | Boise......Idaho | 12. | Evansville......Indiana |
| 13. | Keokuk......Iowa | 14. | Decatur....Illinois Indiana Georgia |
| 15. | Wichita......Kansas | 16. | Louisville......Kentucky |
| 17. | Baton Rouge......Louisiana | 18. | Bangor......Maine |
| 19. | Annapolis......Maryland | 20. | Boston......Massachusetts |
| 21. | Holland......Michigan | 22. | St. Paul......Minnesota |
| 23. | Bullock......Mississippi | 24. | Butte......Montana |
| 25. | Branson......Missouri | 26. | Lincoln......Illinois Nebraska |
| 27. | Utica......New York | 28. | Trenton......New Jersey |
| 29. | Santa Fe......New Mexico | 30. | Concord......New Hampshire |
| 31. | Charlotte......North Carolina | 32. | Bismarck......Illinois North Dakota |
| 33. | Akron......Ohio | 34. | Enid......Oklahoma |
| 35. | Madison......Wisconsin | 36. | Nashville......Indiana Tennessee |
| 37. | Richmond......Virginia | 38. | Charleston......Illinois S. Carolina |
| 39. | Cheyenne......Wyoming | 40. | Tacoma......Washington |
| 41. | Montpelier......Vermont | 42. | Austin......Texas |

# TWO CITIES - YOU NAME THE STATE
CREATED BY GLENN SEYMOUR

1. Yuma & Flagstaff _____

2. Salem & Portland _____

3. Ypsilanti & Holland _____

4. Queens & Syracuse _____

5. Beaver & Wausau _____

6. Waco & Austin _____

7. Anchorage & Juneau _____

8. Orlando & Miami _____

9. Santa Fe & Gallop _____

10. Honolulu & Pearl Harbor _____

11. Springfield & Zion _____

12. Columbus & Cincinnati _____

13. Spokane & Seattle _____

14. Provo & Salt Lake City _____

15. Little Rock & Fort Smith _____

16. Evansville & South Bend _____

17. Birmingham & Huntsville _____

18. Boise & Pocatello _____

19. Wilmington & Dover _____

20. Burlington & Montpelier _____

21. Los Angeles & Apple Valley _____

22. Boulder & Fort Collins _____

23. Waterbury & New Haven _____

24. Augusta & Albany _____

25. Sioux City & Cedar Rapids _____

26. Wichita & Topeka _____

27. Bowling Green & Corbin _____

28. North Platte & Omaha _____

29. Yellowstone & Cheyenne _____

30. Meridian & Biloxi _____

31. Fayette & Wilmington _____

32. Bismarck & Fargo _____

33. Helena & Butte _____

34. Tulsa & Enid _____

35. Concord & Manchester _____

36. Las Vegas & Reno _____

37. Wheeling & Charleston _____

38. Hagerstown & Annapolis _____

39. Newport & Providence _____

40. Rochester & Stipule _____

41. Atlantic City & Trenton _____

42. Memphis & Saratoga _____

43. Erie & Philadelphia _____

44. Columbia & Greenville _____

# TWO CITIES - YOU NAME THE STATE
## CREATED BY GLENN SEYMOUR

1. Yuma & Flagstaff.............................. Arizona
2. Salem & Portland................................Oregon
3. Ypsilanti & Holland...................... Michigan
4. Queens & Syracuse..........................New York
5. Beaver & Wausau..........................Wisconsin
6. Waco & Austin ....................................... Texas
7. Anchorage & Juneau ......................... Alaska
8. Orlando & Miami .............................. Florida
9. Santa Fe & Gallop ..................... New Mexico
10. Honolulu & Pearl Harbor ...................Hawaii
11. Springfield & Zion ..............................Illinois
12. Columbus & Cincinnati..........................Ohio
13. Spokane & Seattle ...................... Washington
14. Provo & Salt Lake City ........................... Utah
15. Little Rock & Fort Smith................ Arkansas
16. Evansville & South Bend ....................Indiana
17. Birmingham & Huntsville ............. Alabama
18. Boise & Pocatello .................................Idaho
19. Wilmington & Dover .....................Delaware
20. Burlington & Montpelier ................ Vermont
21. Los Angeles & Apple Valley ........ California
22. Boulder & Fort Collins ................... Colorado
23. Waterbury & New Haven ......... Connecticut
24. Augusta & Albany............................... Georgia
25. Sioux City & Cedar Rapids....................Iowa
26. Wichita & Topeka ...............................Kansas
27. Bowling Green & Corbin...............Kentucky
28. North Platte & Omaha ....................Nebraska
29. Yellowstone & Cheyenne .............. Wyoming
30. Meridian & Biloxi ........................Mississippi
31. Fayette & Wilmington.......... North Carolina
32. Bismarck & Fargo .....................North Dakota
33. Helena & Butte................................. Montana
34. Tulsa& Enid .................................. Oklahoma
35. Concord & Manchester.......New Hampshire
36. Las Vegas & Reno ...............................Nevada
37. Wheeling & Charleston .......... West Virginia
38. Hagerstown & Annapolis ...............Maryland
39. Newport & Providence .......... Massachusetts
40. Rochester & Stipule .......................Minnesota
41. Atlantic City & Trenton ..............New Jersey
42. Memphis & Saratoga ......................Tennessee
43. Erie & Philadelphia ................. Pennsylvania
44. Columbia & Greenville ......... South Carolina

# ITEMS CONNECTED WITH STATE, COUNTRY, ETC.

CREATED BY GLENN SEYMOUR

1.  Rodeo City _____

2.  Islands _____

3.  Grand Ole Opry _____

4.  Lone Star State _____

5.  Painted Desert _____

6.  Disney World _____

7.  Chocolate City _____

8.  Land of Lincoln _____

9.  Peach State _____

10. White Sands _____

11. Land of 1000 Lakes _____

12. Grand Canyon _____

13. Blue Ridge Mountains _____

14. Mardi Gras _____

15. Keys _____

16. Silver Dollar City _____

17. Palm Beach _____

18. Gambling State _____

# ITEMS CONNECTED WITH STATE, COUNTRY, ETC.
CREATED BY GLENN SEYMOUR

1.  Rodeo City ........................................................................................................................... Cheyenne

2.  Islands .................................................................................................................................. Canary

3.  Grand Ole Opry .................................................................................................................. Nashville

4.  Lone Star State .................................................................................................................... Texas

5.  Painted Desert .................................................................................................................... Arizona

6.  Disney World ....................................................................................................................... Florida

7.  Chocolate City .................................................................................................................... Hershey

8.  Land of Lincoln .................................................................................................................. Illinois

9.  Peach State .......................................................................................................................... Georgia

10. White Sands ........................................................................................................................ New Mexico

11. Land of 1000 Lakes ............................................................................................................ Minnesota

12. Grand Canyon ..................................................................................................................... Arizona

13. Blue Ridge Mountains ....................................................................................................... Virginia

14. Mardi Gras .......................................................................................................................... New Orleans

15. Keys ...................................................................................................................................... Florida

16. Silver Dollar City ............................................................................................................... Missouri

17. Palm Beach .......................................................................................................................... Florida

18. Gambling State .................................................................................................................... Nevada

# STATES & CITIES IN SONGS

CREATED BY GLENN SEYMOUR

1. Come From _____ With my Banjo on my Knee

2. The Sidewalks of _____

3. _____Moon Keep Shining

4. _____ Jubilee

5. The Blue Ridge Mountains of _____

6. Moon Over _____

7. _____Mud

8. _____ Choo Choo

9. By The River Gently Flowin _____

10. _____ Waltz

11. Beautiful _____

12. My Old _____Home

13. I Left My Heart In _____

14. Battle of _____

15. White Cliffs of _____

16. _____ Cannonball

17. Meet Me In _____

18. Back Home In _____

19. _____ Here I Come

20. _____ Traveler

# STATES & CITIES IN SONGS
### CREATED BY GLENN SEYMOUR

1. Come From ..........................Alabama..................With my Banjo on my Knee

2. The Sidewalks of ...........................New York ..............................................

3. ................................................Carolina ........................... Moon Keep  Shining

4. ................................................Alabama........................................Jubilee

5. The Blue Ridge Moutains of...........Virginia .......................................................

6. Moon Over.............................Miami.....................................................

7. ................................................Mississippi .......................................Mud

8. ................................................Chattanooga.....................................Choo Choo

9. By The River Gently Flowing...........Illinois ...................................................

10. ................................................Missouri - Tennessee ............................... Waltz

11. Beautiful ................................Ohio ....................................................

12. My Old...............................Kentucky...................................Home

13. I Left My Heart In .........................San Francisco .......................................

14. Battle of...............................New Orleans ........................................

15. White Cliffs of...............................Dover  .......................................

16. ................................................Wabash...............................Cannonball

17. Meet Me In ...........................St. Louie .........................................

18. Back Home In ...........................Indiana.........................................

19. ................................................California........................Here I Come

20. ................................................ Arkansas ................................ Traveler

# UNITED STATES

CREATED BY GLENN SEYMOUR

| | STATE | CAPITOL | STATE FLOWER | STATE BIRD |
|---|---|---|---|---|
| 1. | Alabama | | | |
| 2. | Alaska | | | |
| 3. | Arizona | | | |
| 4. | Arkansas | | | |
| 5. | California | | | |
| 6. | Colorado | | | |
| 7. | Connecticut | | | |
| 8. | Delaware | | | |
| 9. | Florida | | | |
| 10. | Georgia | | | |
| 11. | Hawaii | | | |
| 12. | Idaho | | | |
| 13. | Illinois | | | |
| 14. | Indiana | | | |
| 15. | Iowa | | | |
| 16. | Kansas | | | |
| 17. | Kentucky | | | |
| 18. | Louisiana | | | |
| 19. | Maine | | | |
| 20. | Maryland | | | |
| 21. | Massachusetts | | | |
| 22. | Michigan | | | |
| 23. | Minnesota | | | |
| 24. | Mississippi | | | |
| 25. | Missouri | | | |
| 26. | Montana | | | |

# UNITED STATES
CREATED BY GLENN SEYMOUR

| | STATE | CAPITOL | STATE FLOWER | STATE BIRD |
|---|---|---|---|---|
| 27. | Nebraska ........... | | | |
| 28. | Nevada ............. | | | |
| 29. | New Hampshire | | | |
| 30. | New Jersey ........ | | | |
| 31. | New Mexico...... | | | |
| 32. | New York ......... | | | |
| 33. | North Carolina. | | | |
| 34. | North Dakota ... | | | |
| 35. | Ohio.................. | | | |
| 36. | Oklahoma ........ | | | |
| 37. | Oregon ............. | | | |
| 38. | Pennsylvania..... | | | |
| 39. | Rhode Island .... | | | |
| 40. | South Carolina . | | | |
| 41. | South Dakota.... | | | |
| 42. | Tennessee ......... | | | |
| 43. | Texas................. | | | |
| 44. | Utah.................. | | | |
| 45. | Vermont........... | | | |
| 46. | Virginia ............. | | | |
| 47. | Washington....... | | | |
| 48. | West Virginia.... | | | |
| 49. | Wisconsin ........ | | | |
| 50. | Wyoming .......... | | | |

# UNITED STATES
## CREATED BY GLENN SEYMOUR

|     | STATE | CAPITOL | STATE FLOWER | STATE BIRD |
| --- | --- | --- | --- | --- |
| 1. | Alabama | Montgomery | Camellia | Yellow Hammer |
| 2. | Alaska | Juneau | Forget Me Not | Willow Ptarmigan |
| 3. | Arizona | Pheoniz | Saguaro Catcus | Cactus Wren |
| 4. | Arkansas | Little Rock | Apple Blossom | Mockingbird |
| 5. | California | Sacramento | Golden Poppy | Cal Valley Quail |
| 6. | Colorado | Denver | Columbine | Lark Bunting |
| 7. | Connecticut | Harford | Mountain Laurel | Robin |
| 8. | Delaware | Dover | Peach Blossom | Blue Hen Chicken |
| 9. | Florida | Tallahassee | Orange Blossom | Mockingbird |
| 10. | Georgia | Atlanta | Cherokee Rose | Brown Thrush |
| 11. | Hawaii | Honolulu | Yellow Hibiscus | Goose |
| 12. | Idaho | Boise | Syringa | Mountain Bluebird |
| 13. | Illinois | Springfield | Violet | Cardinal |
| 14. | Indiana | Indianapolis | Peony | Cardinal |
| 15. | Iowa | DesMoines | Wild Rose | Eastern Golden Finch |
| 16. | Kansas | Topeka | Sunflower | Western Meadowlark |
| 17. | Kentucky | Frankfort | Golden Rod | Cardinal |
| 18. | Louisiana | Baton Rouge | Mongolia | Eastern Brown Pelican |
| 19. | Maine | Augusta | Pine Cone Tassel | Chickadee |
| 20. | Maryland | Annapolis | Black Eyed Susan | Baltimore Oriole |
| 21. | Massachusetts | Boston | Mayflower | Chickadee |
| 22. | Michigan | Lansing | Apple Blossom | Robin |
| 23. | Minnesota | St. Paul | Lady Slipper | Common Loon |
| 24. | Mississippi | Jackson | Magnolia | Mocking Bird |
| 25. | Missouri | Jefferson City | Hawthorn | Bluebird |
| 26. | Montana | Helena | Bitterroot | Western Meadowlark |

# UNITED STATES
## CREATED BY GLENN SEYMOUR

| | STATE | CAPITOL | STATE FLOWER | STATE BIRD |
|---|---|---|---|---|
| 27. | Nebraska | Lincoln | Goldenrod | Western Meadowlark |
| 28. | Nevada | Carson City | Sagebrush | Mountain Bluebird |
| 29. | New Hampshire | Concord | Purple Lilac | Purple Finch |
| 30. | New Jersey | Trenton | Violet | Eastern Goldfinch |
| 31. | New Mexico | Santa Fe | Yucca | Roadrunner |
| 32. | New York | Albany | Rose | Bluebird |
| 33. | North Carolina | Raleigh | Dogwood | Cardinal |
| 34. | North Dakota | Bismarck | Wild Prairie Rose | Western Meadowlark |
| 35. | Ohio | Columbus | Scarlet Carnation | Cardinal |
| 36. | Oklahoma | Oklahoma City | Mistletoe | Scissor Tail Fly Catcher |
| 37. | Oregon | Salem | Oregon Grape | Western Meadowlark |
| 38. | Pennsylvania | Harrisburg | Mountain Laurel | Ruffed Grouse |
| 39. | Rhode Island | Providence | Violet | Rhode Island Red |
| 40. | South Carolina | Columbia | Yellow Jessamine | Great Carolina Wren |
| 41. | South Dakota | Pierre | Pasqual Flower | Ring Tail Pheasant |
| 42. | Tennessee | Nashville | Iris | Mockingbird |
| 43. | Texas | Austin | Bluebonnet | Mockingbird |
| 44. | Utah | Salt Lake City | Sego Lily | Common American Gull |
| 45. | Vermont | Montpellier | Dogwood | Hermit Thrush |
| 46. | Virginia | Richmond | Willow Goldfish | Pink Rhododendron |
| 47. | Washington | Charleston | Pink Rhododendron | Willow Goldfinch |
| 48. | West Virginia | Charleston | Rhododendron | Cardinal |
| 49. | Wisconsin | Madison | Wood Violet | Robin |
| 50. | Wyoming | Cheyenne | Indian Paintbrush | Western Meadowlark |

# STATES WITH VOWELS MISSING

## CREATED BY GLENN SEYMOUR

1. _ l _ b _ m _ _____

2. C _ l _ f _ rn _ _ _____

3. D _ l _ w _ r _ _____

4. _ l _ sk _ _____

5. _ r _ z _ n _ _____

6. C _ l _ r _ d _ _____

7. _ _ w _ _____

8. _ rk _ ns _ s _____

9. C _ nn _ ct _ c _ t _____

10. H _ w _ _ _ _____

11. G _ _ rg _ _ _____

12. _ d _ h _ _____

13. K _ ns _ s _____

14. _ ll _ n _ _ s _____

15. L _ _ _ s _ _ n _ _____

16. _ nd _ _ n _ _____

17. K _ nt _ cky _____

18. M _ _ n _ _____

19. N _ br _ sk _ _____

20. M _ ryl _ nd _____

21. M _ ss _ ss _ pp _ _____

22. N _ v _ d _ _____

23. M _ ss _ ch _ s _ tts _____

24. N _ w M _ x _ c _ _____

25. M _ ch _ g _ n _____

26. M _ ss _ _ r _ _____

27. N _ w J _ rs _ y _____

28. M _ nn _ s _ t _ _____

29. N _ w Y _ rk _____

30. M _ nt _ n _ _____

31. N _ rth C _ r _ l _ n _ _____

32. _ h _ _ _____

33. N _ rth D _ k _ t _ _____

34. _ r _ g _ n _____

35. P _ nnsylv _ n _ _ _____

36. _ kl _ h _ m _ _____

37. Rh _ d _ _ sl _ nd _____

38. S _ _ th C _ r _ l _ n _ _____

39. T _ nn _ ss _ _ _____

40. S _ _ th D _ k _ t _ _____

41. T _ x _ s _____

42. _ t _ h _____

43. V _ rm _ nt _____

44. W _ sh _ ngt _ n _____

45. V _ rg _ n _ _ _____

46. Fl _ r _ d _ _____

47. W _ st V _ rg _ n _ _ _____

48. W _ sc _ ns _ n _____

49. Wy _ m _ ng _____

50. N _ w H _ mpsh _ r _ _____

# STATES WITH VOWELS MISSING
CREATED BY GLENN SEYMOUR

1. _ l _ b _ m _ ............................ Alabama
2. C _ l _ f _ rn _ _ .................... California
3. D _ l _ w _ r _ ......................... Delaware
4. _ l _ sk _ .................................... Alaska
5. _ r _ z _ n _ .............................. Arizona
6. C _ l _ r _ d _ ......................... Colorado
7. _ _ w _ ......................................... Iowa
8. _ rk _ ns _ s ........................... Arkansas
9. C _ nn _ ct _ c _ t .............. Connecticut
10. H _ w _ _ _ ................................. Hawaii
11. G _ _ rg _ _ ............................... Georgia
12. _ d _ h _ ...................................... Idaho
13. K _ ns _ s .................................. Kansas
14. _ ll _ n _ _ s ................................ Illinois
15. L _ _ _ s _ _ n _ ..................... Louisiana
16. _ nd _ _ n _ ............................. Indiana
17. K _ nt _ cky ........................... Kentucky
18. M _ _ n _ .................................... Maine
19. N _ br _ sk _ ............................ Nebraska
20. M _ ryl _ nd ........................... Maryland
21. M _ ss _ ss _ pp _ ................. Mississippi
22. N _ v _ d _ ................................. Nevada
23. M _ ss _ ch _ s _ tts ......... Massachusetts
24. N _ w M _ x _ c _ ............... New Mexico
25. M _ ch _ g _ n ......................... Michigan

26. M _ ss _ _ r _ ........................... Missouri
27. N _ w J _ rs _ y ..................... New Jersey
28. M _ nn _ s _ t _ .................... Minnesota
29. N _ w Y _ rk .......................... New York
30. M _ nt _ n _ ........................... Montana
31. N _ rth C _ r _ l _ n _ ... North Carolina
32. _ h _ _ .......................................... Ohio
33. N _ rth D _ k _ t _ ........... North Dakota
34. _ r _ g _ n .................................. Oregon
35. P _ nnsylv _ n _ _ .............. Pennsylvania
36. _ kl _ h _ m _ ....................... Oklahoma
37. Rh _ d _ _ sl _ nd ........... Rhode Island
38. S _ _ th C _ r _ l _ n _ ....South Carolina
39. T _ nn _ ss _ _ ...................... Tennessee
40. S _ _ th D _ k _ t _ .......... South Dakota
41. T _ x _ s ...................................... Texas
42. _ t _ h ......................................... Utah
43. V _ rm _ nt .............................. Vermont
44. W _ sh _ ngt _ n .................. Washington
45. V _ rg _ n _ _ ........................... Virginia
46. Fl _ r _ d _ .................................. Florida
47. W _ st V _ rg _ n _ _ ......... West Virginia
48. W _ sc _ ns _ n ...................... Wisconsin
49. Wy _ m _ ng ........................... Wyoming
50. N _ w H _ mpsh _ r _ . New Hampshire

# WHAT STATE IS THIS CITY IN?
## (Most of these are NOT capitals)
CREATED BY GLENN SEYMOUR

1. Nome _____

2. Yuma _____

3. Little Rock _____

4. Mobile _____

5. Denver _____

6. Hartford _____

7. Orlando _____

8. Dover _____

9. Macon _____

10. Honolulu _____

11. Boise _____

12. Evansville _____

13. Keokuk _____

14. Decatur _____

15. Wichita _____

16. Louisville _____

17. Baton Rouge _____

18. Bangor _____

19. Annapolis _____

20. Boston _____

21. Holland _____

22. St. Paul _____

23. Bullock _____

24. Butte _____

25. Branson _____

26. Lincoln _____

27. Utica _____

28. Trenton _____

29. Santa Fe _____

30. Concord _____

31. Charlotte _____

32. Bismarck _____

33. Akron _____

34. Enid _____

35. Madison _____

36. Nashville _____

37. Richmond _____

38. Cheyenne _____

39. Tacoma _____

40. Montpelier _____

# WHAT STATE IS THIS CITY IN?
## (Most of these are NOT capitals)
CREATED BY GLENN SEYMOUR

1. Nome............................Alaska
2. Yuma ........................ Arizona
3. Little Rock......................... Arkansas
4. Mobile ................................Alabama
5. Denver................................Colorado
6. Hartford.........................Connecticut
7. Orlando....................................Florida
8. Dover....Delaware - New Hampshire
9. Macon ...................................... Georgia
10. Honolulu.................................Hawaii
11. Boise ...........................................Idaho
12. Evansville...............................Indiana
13. Keokuk.........................................Iowa
14. Decatur.. Illinois - Indiana - Georgia
15. Wichita........................................Kansas
16. Louisville..........................Kentucky
17. Baton Rouge ...................... Louisiana
18. Bangor ................................ Maine
19. Annapolis.......................... Maryland
20. Boston ...................... Massachusetts

21. Holland ...............................Michigan
22. St. Paul..............................Minnesota
23. Bullock ..............................Mississippi
24. Butte ........................................Montana
25. Branson ...............................Missouri
26. Lincoln ................. Illinois- Nebraska
27. Utica ................................... New York
28. Trenton............................New Jersey
29. Santa Fe ......................... New Mexico
30. Concord ..................New Hampshire
31. Charlotte .................. North Carolina
32. Bismarck ...... Illinois - North Dakota
33. Akron ........................................ Ohio
34. Enid ................................Oklahoma
35. Madison ...........................Wisconsin
36. Nashvllle ...........Indiana - Tennessee
37. Richmond ............................. Virginia
38. Cheyenne............................Wyoming
39. Tacoma...........................Washington
40. Montpelier ...........................Vermont

# MATH

# MATH
## CREATED BY GLENN SEYMOUR

1.  A heater burns 1/2 gallon of oil per hour, how much oil will it burn in 24 hours? _____

2.  I buy 6 candy bars for 10 cents each, get one free. How much do I owe for 7 candy bars? _____

3.  I get 10% discount of $200.00 groceries. How much do I pay? _____

4.  A rabbit runs across a field in 3 minutes. The dog runs 1/2 as fast. How long will it take the dog to run across the field? _____

5.  If you take one pill twice a day, how many pills would you need for 90 days? _____

6.  Pop is 10 cents a can, 12 pack $1.00. I buy 1 - 12pack and 2 cans. How much do I owe for the pop? _____

7.  Melons are $3.00, reduced 25%. How much for a melon? _____

8.  4 out of every 5 seed of corn grew. What percent stand do I have? _____

9.  Shoes are originally $60.00 a pair, but today they are 50% off. How much is a pair of shoes? _____

10. A car uses 1 pint of oil in 600 miles. How many miles do I drive before I have to add a quart? _____

11. I need 1 1/2 gallons of antifreeze at $4.50 a gallon. How much do I owe? _____

12. If pay a $300.00 seed corn bill on time, I get 5% discount. How much will I pay? _____ How much do I save? _____

13. If I pay a $35.00 telephone bill, the late fine is 10%. How much do I have to pay? _____

14. I pay $20.00 per acre and 3 cents a bushel to combine one acre and 150 bushel of corn. How much do I pay? _____

15. Cows are 40 cents a pound. How much for a 225 pound cow? _____

16. 3 1/2 yards of material at $3.00 per yard is? _____

17. An airplane averages 600 miles per hour . How far would it go in 6 hours? _____

18. A seamstress charges $6.00 per hour . If she works 3 hours how much will she make? _____

19. The first cup of coffee is 40 cents, all others are 15 cents. I drink 3 cups. How much do I owe for the coffee? _____

20. A book has 240 pages . I read 40 pages a day. How long will it take me to read this book ? _____

21. If I type 100 words a minute. How long will it take me to type 2500 words? _____

# MATH
## CREATED BY GLENN SEYMOUR

1. A heater burns 1/2 gallon of oil per hour, how much oil will it burn in 24 hours? ......................................................................................... 12 gallon

2. I buy 6 candy bars for 10 cents each, get one free. How much do I owe for 7 candy bars? ......................................................................................... 60 cents

3. I get 10% discount of $200.00 groceries. How much do I pay? ......................... $180.00

4. A rabbit runs across a field in 3 minutes. The dog runs 1/2 as fast. How long will it take the dog to run across the field? ............................................. 6 minutes

5. If you take one pill twice a day, how many pills would you need for 90 days? ......................................................................................................... 180

6. Pop is 10 cents a can, 12 pack $1.00. I buy 1 - 12pack and 2 cans. How much do I owe for the pop? ................................................................................ $1.20

7. Melons are $3.00, reduced 25%. How much for a melon? ................................. $2.25

8. 4 out of every 5 seed of corn grew. What percent stand do I have? ................. 80%

9. Shoes are originally $60.00 a pair, but today they are 50% off. How much is a pair of shoes? .......................................................................................... $30.00

10. A car uses 1 pint of oil in 600 miles. How many miles do I drive before I have to add a quart? ............................................................................... 1200 miles

11. I need 1 1/2 gallons of antifreeze at $4.50 a gallon. How much do I owe? ........ $6.75

12. If I pay a $300.00 seed corn bill on time, I get 5% discount. How much will I pay? ...................... $285.00 ..... How much do I save? ............................... $15.00

13. If I pay a $35.00 telephone bill, the late fine is 10%. How much do I have to pay? ................................................................................................... $38.50

14. I pay $20.00 per acre and 3 cents a bushel to combine one acre and 150 bushel of corn. How much do I pay? ...................................................................... $24.50

15. Cows are 40 cents a pound. How much for a 225 pound cow? ......................... $90.00

16. 3 1/2 yards of material at $3.00 per yard is? ...................................................... $10.50

17. An airplane averages 600 miles per hour . How far would it go in 6 hours? . 3600 m

18. A seamstress charges $6.00 per hour . If she works 3 hours how much will she make? ................................................................................................... $18.00

19. The first cup of coffee is 40 cents, all others are 15 cents. I drink 3 cups. How much do I owe for the coffee? ................................................................ 70 cents

20. A book has 240 pages . I read 40 pages a day. How long will it take me to read this book ? ................................................................................................... 6 days

21. If I type 100 words a minute. How long will it take me to type 2500 words? . 25 min.

# WEIGHTS & MEASURES
## CREATED BY GLENN SEYMOUR

1.   How many inches in a foot? _____

2.   What is the abbreviation for foot? _____

3.   Name something sold by the foot. _____

4.   How many feet in a yard? _____

5.   How many inches in a yard? _____

6.   What is the abbreviation for yard? _____

7.   How many feet in a rod? _____

8.   How many yards in a rod? _____

9.   Name something sold by the rod. _____

10.  How many ounces in a cup? _____

11.  How many cups in a pint? _____

12.  What is the abbreviation for pint? _____

13.  How many ounces in a pint? _____

14.  Name something sold by the pint._____

15.  How many pints in a quart? _____

16.  What is the abbreviation for quart? _____

17.  Name something sold by the quart. _____

18.  How many quarts in a gallon? _____

19.  What is the abbreviation for gallon? _____

20.  Name something sold by the gallon. _____

21.  How many pounds in a peck? _____

22.  What is the abbreviation for peck? _____

23.  Name something sold by the peck. _____

24.  How many pecks in a bushel? _____

25.  What is the abbreviation for bushel? _____

26.  Name something sold by the bushel. _____

27.  How many pounds in a ton? _____

28.  Name something sold by the ton. _____

# WEIGHTS & MEASURES
## CREATED BY GLENN SEYMOUR

1.  How many inches in a foot? ........................................................................ 12
2.  What is the abbreviation for foot? ............................................................ FT
3.  Name something sold by the foot. ...................................................... LUMBER
4.  How many feet in a yard? ............................................................................ 3
5.  How many inches in a yard? ...................................................................... 36
6.  What is the abbreviation for yard? ............................................................ YD
7.  How many feet in a rod? ...................................................................... 16 ½
8.  How many yards in a rod? ...................................................................... 5 ½
9.  Name something sold by the rod. ....................................................... FENCE
10. How many ounces in a cup? ...................................................................... 8
11. How many cups in a pint? .......................................................................... 2
12. What is the abbreviation for pint? ............................................................ PT
13. How many ounces in a pint? .................................................................... 16
14. Name something sold by the pint. ......................................................... MILK
15. How many pints in a quart? ...................................................................... 2
16. What is the abbreviation for quart? ......................................................... QT
17. Name something sold by the quart. ............................................... ICE CREAM
18. How many quarts in a gallon? .................................................................... 4
19. What is the abbreviation for gallon? ....................................................... GAL
20. Name something sold by the gallon ...................................................... PAINT
21. How many pounds in a peck? .................................................................. 15
22. What is the abbreviation for peck? .......................................................... PK
23. Name something sold by the peck. ..................................................... APPLES
24. How many pecks in a bushel? .................................................................... 4
25. What is the abbreviation for bushel? ........................................................ BU
26. Name something sold by the bushel. ................................................. PEACHES
27. How many pounds in a ton? ................................................................. 2000
28. Name something sold by the ton. .......................................................... COAL

# GROCERY SHOPPING
## CREATED BY GLENN SEYMOUR

1. Bananas $.30 a pound , over ripe, half price - how much are the over ripe bananas _____

2. Apples two pounds $.25 - how much are 4 pounds? _____

3. Hamburger one dollar a pound - how much is 1 and ½ pounds of hamburger_____

4. Cookies two for quarter - how much is six cookies? _____

5. Milk is $3.00 per gallon - how much is a quart?_____

6. Buy two pounds of apples, get one free apple, - if you buy 8 pounds of apples how many free apples do you get? _____

7. Four grapefruit cost $1.00 - there are only three grapefruit. How much does the grapefruit cost?_____

8. Salt cost $.03 an ounce - how much is one pound of salt? _____

9. I buy one pound of hamburger $1.00, one package of buns 75 cents, one loaf of bread $1.00, then decide to put the bread back - how much do I owe? _____

10. Fifteen pounds of potatoes at $.10 a pound is _____

11. Purchased a bushel of peaches at $9.50, the refund for returning basket is $1.00. How much did the peaches cost? _____

12. Antifreeze is $12.00 for 24 quarts. How much is one quart? _____

13. I buy 2 pies, one cost $2.50, the other one cost $2.75. Gave the clerk $5.00. What is wrong? _____

14. I buy one box of Wheaties for $3.75. Gave the clerk $5.00. How much change do I get back?_____

15. Ice cream is $5.00 a gallon. How much is a quart? _____

16. One pint of Half and Half is $.49. How much is a quart?_____

17. I buy 4 peppers for $1.00, one package of carrots for $.75, one package of Onions for $.15. How much do I owe? _____

18. I buy 5 bottles of pop at $.25 each, returned one bottle for $.05. How much more do I owe? _____

19. Four packages of cookies cost $1.50 a package, gave the clerk $5.00. How Much more do I owe? _____

20. Two T-bone steaks cost $3.50, how much is one steak? _____

21. A bushel of potatoes is $3.50, how much is a peck? _____

22. Canned corn is 3 for $.80, bought 6 cans, how much do I owe? _____

23. Canned peaches are $1.25 a can, bought 4 cans, how much do I owe? _____

24. Cookies are $.12 each, bought 4, how much do I owe? _____

25. Sliced turkey is $3.00 a pound , how much can I get for $6.00_____

# GROCERY SHOPPING
## CREATED BY GLENN SEYMOUR

1. Bananas $.30 a pound , over ripe, half price - how much are the over ripe bananas.... $.15 per pound

2. Apples two pounds $.25 - how much are 4 pounds? .................................................. $.50

3. Hamburger one dollar a pound - how much is 1 and ½ pounds of hamburger.......... $1.50

4. Cookies two for quarter - how much is six cookies? ................................................ $.75

5. Milk is $3.00 per gallon - how much is a quart?...................................................... $.75

6. Buy two pounds of apples, get one free apple, - if you buy 8 pounds of apples how many free apples do you get? ..................................................................... 4 Apples

7. Four grapefruit cost $1.00 - there are only three grapefruit. How much does the grapefruit cost? ....................................................................................... $.75

8. Salt cost $.03 an ounce - how much is one pound of salt? ........................................ $.24

9. I buy one pound of hamburger $1.00, one package of buns 75 cents, one loaf of bread $1.00, then decide to put the bread back - how much do I owe? ................. $1.75

10. Fifteen pounds of potatoes at $.10 a pound is ......................................................... $1.50

11. Purchased a bushel of peaches at $9.50, the refund for returning basket is $1.00. How much did the peaches cost? .......................................................... $8.50

12. Antifreeze is $12.00 for 24 quarts. How much is one quart? .................................. $.50

13. I buy 2 pies, one cost $2.50, the other one cost $2.75. Gave the clerk $5.00. What is wrong?.......................................................................... owe the clerk $.25

14. I buy one box of Wheaties for $3.75. Gave the clerk $5.00. How much change do I get back?........................................................................................................ $1.25

15. Ice cream is $5.00 a gallon. How much is a quart?................................................. $1.25

16. One pint of Half and Half is $.49. How much is a quart?...................................... $.98

17. I buy 4 peppers for $1.00, one package of carrots for $.75, one package of Onions for $.15. How much do I owe? ............................................................................ $1.90

18. I buy 5 bottles of pop at $.25 each, returned one bottle for $.05. How much more do I owe?............................................................................................................ $1.20

19. Four packages of cookies cost $1.50 a package, gave the clerk $5.00. How Much more do I owe?.................................................................................................... $1.00

20. Two T-bone steaks cost $3.50, how much is one steak? ......................................... $1.75

21. A bushel of potatoes is $3.50, how much is a peck?.............................................. $1.00

22. Canned corn is 3 for $.80, bought 6 cans, how much do I owe?............................ $1.60

23. Canned peaches are $1.25  a can, bought 4 cans, how much do I owe?................. $5.00

24. Cookies are $.12 each, bought 4, how much do I owe?.......................................... $.48

25. Sliced turkey is $3.00 a pound , how much can I get for $6.00........................ 2 pounds

# MATH
## CREATED BY GLENN SEYMOUR

1. $3 + 3 + 5 =$ _____

2. $5 + 0 + 5 =$ _____

3. $9 + 4 =$ _____

4. $13 - 6 =$ _____

5. $13 + 7 =$ _____

6. $10 - 0 + 1 =$ _____

7. $4 + 4 + 4 =$ _____

8. $7 + 8 =$ _____

9. $20 - 9 =$ _____

10. $22 + 11 =$ _____

11. $16 + 4 =$ _____

12. $5 + 4 - 3 =$ _____

13. $12 + 3 - 5 =$ _____

14. $4 + 4 - 8 =$ _____

15. $5 + 0 =$ _____

16. $2 \times 11 =$ _____

17. $2 \times 8 =$ _____

18. $3 \times 7 =$ _____

19. $5 \times 5 =$ _____

20. $2 \times 2 \times 2 =$ _____

21. $8 \times 8 =$ _____

22. $10 \times 10 =$ _____

23. $4 \times 7 =$ _____

24. $10 \times 10 \times 5 =$ _____

25. $8 \div 4 =$ _____

26. $15 \div 3 =$ _____

27. $20 \div 4 =$ _____

28. $21 \div 3 =$ _____

29. $33 \div 3 =$ _____

30. $75 \div 3 =$ _____

31. $99 \div 11 =$ _____

32. $32 \div 4 =$ _____

33. $49 \div 7 =$ _____

34. $63 \div 3 =$ _____

35. $100 \div 10 =$ _____

36. $5 \div 1 =$ _____

37. $1/2 \div 1/2 =$ _____

38. $1/2 \times 1/2 =$ _____

39. $4 + 1/2 =$ _____

40. $4 - 1/4 =$ _____

41. $3 - 1\ 1/2 =$ _____

42. $5 \div 2 =$ _____

43. $1/2 + 1/2 + 1/2 =$ _____

44. $1/3 + 2/3 =$ _____

45. $3/4 + 3/4 =$ _____

46. $2 - 1/4 =$ _____

# MATH
## CREATED BY GLENN SEYMOUR

| | | |
|---|---|---|
| 1. | $3 + 3 + 5 =$ ..................................... 11 | |
| 2. | $5 + 0 + 5 =$ ..................................... 10 | |
| 3. | $9 + 4 =$ ..................................... 13 | |
| 4. | $13 - 6 =$ ..................................... 7 | |
| 5. | $13 + 7 =$ ..................................... 20 | |
| 6. | $10 - 0 + 1 =$ ..................................... 11 | |
| 7. | $4 + 4 + 4 =$ ..................................... 12 | |
| 8. | $7 + 8 =$ ..................................... 15 | |
| 9. | $20 - 9 =$ ..................................... 11 | |
| 10. | $22 + 11 =$ ..................................... 33 | |
| 11. | $16 + 4 =$ ..................................... 20 | |
| 12. | $5 + 4 - 3 =$ ..................................... 6 | |
| 13. | $12 + 3 - 5 =$ ..................................... 10 | |
| 14. | $4 + 4 - 8 =$ ..................................... 0 | |
| 15. | $5 + 0 =$ ..................................... 5 | |
| 16. | $2 \times 11 =$ ..................................... 22 | |
| 17. | $2 \times 8 =$ ..................................... 16 | |
| 18. | $3 \times 7 =$ ..................................... 21 | |
| 19. | $5 \times 5 =$ ..................................... 25 | |
| 20. | $2 \times 2 \times 2 =$ ..................................... 8 | |
| 21. | $8 \times 8 =$ ..................................... 64 | |
| 22. | $10 \times 10 =$ ..................................... 100 | |
| 23. | $4 \times 7 =$ ..................................... 28 | |

| | |
|---|---|
| 24. | $10 \times 10 \times 5 =$ ..................................... 500 |
| 25. | $8 \div 4 =$ ..................................... 2 |
| 26. | $15 \div 3 =$ ..................................... 5 |
| 27. | $20 \div 4 =$ ..................................... 5 |
| 28. | $21 \div 3 =$ ..................................... 7 |
| 29. | $33 \div 3 =$ ..................................... 11 |
| 30. | $75 \div 3 =$ ..................................... 25 |
| 31. | $99 \div 11 =$ ..................................... 9 |
| 32. | $32 \div 4 =$ ..................................... 8 |
| 33. | $49 \div 7 =$ ..................................... 7 |
| 34. | $63 \div 3 =$ ..................................... 21 |
| 35. | $100 \div 10 =$ ..................................... 10 |
| 36. | $5 \div 1 =$ ..................................... 5 |
| 37. | $1/2 \div 1/2 =$ ..................................... 0 |
| 38. | $1/2 \times 1/2 =$ ..................................... 1 |
| 39. | $4 + 1/2 =$ ..................................... 4 ½ |
| 40. | $4 - 1/4 =$ ..................................... 3 ¾ |
| 41. | $3 - 1 1/2 =$ ..................................... 1 ½ |
| 42. | $5 \div 2 =$ ..................................... 2 ½ |
| 43. | $1/2 + 1/2 + 1/2 =$ ..................................... 1 ½ |
| 44. | $1/3 + 2/3 =$ ..................................... 1 |
| 45. | $3/4 + 3/4 =$ ..................................... 1 ½ |
| 46. | $2 - 1/4 =$ ..................................... 1 ¾ |

# BARGAIN DAY
## CREATED BY GLENN SEYMOUR

1.  Shoes are $50.00 a pair, get one pair ½ price, and one pair 50% off. How much for two pair of shoes? _____

2.  Handkerchiefs are $.40 each, how much for 8? _____

3.  If shoe soles are $2.50 each, heels are $1.50 each, how much would it cost to put soles and heels on a pair of shoes?_____

4.  Washer and dryer at Sears cost $649.00, same washer and dryer cost $849.00 at Penny's. What is the difference? _____

5.  On grocery discount day your total bill is $34.50. The discount if 10%. How much are you saving? _____

6.  Toothpaste is $2.75, toothbrush is $1.75, dental floss is $1.50. How much would all three cost? _____

7.  Bedroom suite is $875.00. With a 10% discount, how would you save? _____

8.  Two cans of hair spray are $9.00. You can get one can free if you buy two. How much would you save on three cans? _____

9.  Yard material is $6.00 a yard, and I want 2 1/3 yards. How much will this cost? ___

10. If you use 2 slices of lunch meat in a sandwich, how many sandwiches will you get out of 18 slices? _____

11. Lace is $.30 a yard, I need 3 ½ yards. How much will it cost?_____

12. Winter coats cost $160.00. They are on sale 25% off. How much will one winter coat cost?_____

13. Tablecloths and napkins are on sale. Tablecloths are $15.00, 4 napkins are $10.00. Today they are 15% off. How much will you pay today for a tablecloth and 4 napkins? _____

14. A lady buys matching shoes and purse. The shoes cost $65.00, the purse is $35.00. They are both 15% off. How much do you pay for a pair of shoes and a purse? _____

# BARGAIN DAY
## CREATED BY GLENN SEYMOUR

1. Shoes are $50.00 a pair, get one pair ½ price, and one pair 50% off. How much for two pair of shoes? ............................................................................................$50.00

2. Handkerchiefs are $.40 each, how much for 8? .......................................$3.20

3. If shoe soles are $2.50 each, heels are $1.50 each, how much would it cost to put soles and heels on a pair of shoes? ........................................................$8.00

4. Washer and dryer at Sears cost $649.00, same washer and dryer cost $849.00 at Penny's. What is the difference? ....................................................$200.00

5. On grocery discount day your total bill is $34.50. The discount if 10%. How much are you saving? ...................................................................................$3.45

6. Toothpaste is $2.75, toothbrush is $1.75, dental floss is $1.50. How much would all three cost? ..............................................................................................$6.00

7. Bedroom suite is $875.00. With a 10% discount, how would you save? ........... $87.50

8. Two cans of hair spray are $9.00. You can get one can free if you buy two. How much would you save on three cans? ..........................................................$3.00

9. Yard material is $6.00 a yard, and I want 2 1/3 yards. How much will this cost? ...... $14.00

10. If you use 2 slices of lunch meat in a sandwich, how many sandwiches will you get out of 18 slices? ...................................................................................... 9

11. Lace is $.30 a yard, I need 3 ½ yards. How much will it cost? ..............................$1.05

12. Winter coats cost $160.00. They are on sale 25% off. How much will one winter coat cost? .........................................................................................$120.00

13. Tablecloths and napkins are on sale. Tablecloths are $15.00, 4 napkins are $10.00. Today they are 15% off. How much will you pay today for a tablecloth and 4 napkins? ....................................................................................................$21.25

14. A lady buys matching shoes and purse. The shoes cost $65.00, the purse is $35.00. They are both 15% off. How much do you pay for a pair of shoes and a purse? ............$85.00

# TIME

CREATED BY GLENN SEYMOUR

1.  How many seconds in a minute? _____

2.  What is 60 minutes? _____

3.  How many minutes in one half hour? _____

4.  How many hours in a day? _____

5.  What is 7 days? _____

6.  How many weeks in a regular February? _____

7.  Which month has 29 days every 4th year? _____

8.  How many days in April? _____

9.  How many days in May? _____

10. How many weeks in a year? _____

11. What is 12 months? _____

12. Which are called summer months? _____

13. Which are called winter months? _____

14. Name a fall month. _____

15. Name a spring month. _____

16. When is the shortest day of the year? _____

17. When is the longest day of the year? _____

18. Name an age in history. _____

19. How many years in a decade? _____

20. How long is a century? _____

21. How many hours in a regular work day? _____

# TIME
## CREATED BY GLENN SEYMOUR

1.  How many seconds in a minute?...................................................................60
2.  What is 60 minutes?................................................................... one hour
3.  How many minutes in one half hour?................................................30
4.  How many hours in a day?.............................................................24
5.  What is 7 days?.............................................................................. week
6.  How many weeks in a regular February?.........................................4
7.  Which month has 29 days every 4th year?..................................... February
8.  How many days in April?..............................................................30
9.  How many days in May?................................................................31
10. How many weeks in a year?..........................................................52
11. What is 12 months?...................................................................1 year
12. Which are called summer months?.................................. June, July, August
13. Which are called winter months?................................... Dec, Jan, Feb
14. Name a fall month......................................................Sept, Oct, Nov
15. Name a spring month. ..........................................March, April, May
16. When is the shortest day of the year?.........................December 21st
17. When is the longest day of the year?............................... June 21st
18. Name an age in history ............................................ stone age, ice age, etc
19. How many years in a decade?.......................................................10
20. How long is a century? ..........................................................100 years
21. How many hours in a regular work day? ........................................8

# MATH
## CREATED BY GLENN SEYMOUR

1. Sweet corn is 4 ears for $1.00. How much for one dozen?_____

2. Play pool for 25 cents a game, 60 cents for 3 games.  I play four  games, how much do I owe? _____

3. It takes 12 pounds of potatoes to plant a row. How many pounds to plant 5 rows? _____

4. A dog eats one pound of feed a puppy 1/4 pound. How much for four dogs and four puppies?_____

5. Hay makes 1 1/2 tons per acre. How much will 10 acres make? _____

6. Two tickets to the show are $5.00. If I buy 5 tickets how much do I owe?  _____

7. If you set 18 tomato plants in a row, how many plants do I need for two rows?_____

8. Tickets to a game are:Adults $2.00, Students 1/2 price.  How much for 3 Adults and 2 Students? _____

9. Hogs are 40 cents a pound.  How much would a 250 pound hog cost?  _____

10. Chicken wire is $1.00 a foot. How much for 4 yards?_____

11. Green onions are 15 cents a dozen. How much for 30 dozen? _____

12. I purchased 150 baby chicks.  10% of them died. How many died? _____

13. A receipe calls for 1 1/4 cups of flour.  If I double it, how much flour do I need to use? _____

14. There are 4 quarts to a gallon. I need 1 3/4 gallon. How many quarts do I need?___

15. If a quart of milk is 65 cents, how much is a gallon?_____

16. If you pick a quart of berries in 10 minutes, how many quarts would you pick in 2 hours? _____

17. I take one pill every 20 minutes. How many do I take in 1 hour :? _____

18. If a well can pump 10 gallons in a minute, how long will it take to pump 500 gallon? _____

19. A carpet is 4 yards wide, 5 yards long. How many square yards? _____

20. A small chain is 12 1/2 cents a foot. How many feet for a dollar?_____

21. If 75 is a passing grade and I answer 15 of 20 questions correctly, do I pass? _____

22. One bag of corn will plant 3 acres, how many bags for 90 acres? _____

23. If I pay my gas bill on time I get 10% off. My bill is $29.00. How much do I get off?_____

24. Of 1000 people, 35% smoke. How many smoke? _____

# MATH
## CREATED BY GLENN SEYMOUR

1. Sweet corn is 4 ears for $1.00. How much for one dozen?...................................$3.00

2. Play pool for 25 cents a game, 60 cents for 3 games. I play four games, how much do I owe?........................................................................................................85 cents

3. It takes 12 pounds of potatoes to plant a row. How many pounds to plant 5 rows?...........................................................................................................60 pounds

4. A dog eats one pound of feed a puppy 1/4 pound. How much for four dogs and four puppies?.....................................................................................................5 pounds

5. Hay makes 1 1/2 tons per acre. How much will 10 acres make?........................15 tons

6. Two tickets to the show are $5.00. If I buy 5 tickets how much do I owe?.......$12.50

7. If you set 18 tomato plants in a row, how many plants do I need for two rows?...........................................................................................................36 plants

8. Tickets to a game are: Adults $2.00, Students 1/2 price. How much for 3 Adults and 2 Students?.........................................................................................................$8.00

9. Hogs are 40 cents a pound. How much would a 250 pound hog cost?.........$100.00

10. Chicken wire is $1.00 a foot. How much for 4 yards?.........................................$12.00

11. Green onions are 15 cents a dozen. How much for 30 dozen?............................$4.50

12. I purchased 150 baby chicks. 10% of them died. How many died?.....15 chicks died

13. A receipe calls for 1 1/4 cups of flour. If I double it, how much flour do I need to use?..............................................................................................................2 ½ cups

14. There are 4 quarts to a gallon. I need 1 3/4 gallon. How many quarts do I need?...........................................................................................................7 quarts

15. If a quart of milk is 65 cents, how much is a gallon?............................................$2.60

16. If you pick a quart of berries in 10 minutes, how many quarts would you pick in 2 hours?............................................................................................................12 quarts

17. I take one pill every 20 minutes. How many do I take in 1 hour :? ...........................3

18. If a well can pump 10 gallons in a minute, how long will it take to pump 500 gallon? .............................................................................................................50 minutes

19. A carpet is 4 yards wide, 5 yards long. How many square yards?............................20

20. A small chain is 12 1/2 cents a foot. How many feet for a dollar? .............................8

21. If 75 is a passing grade and I answer 15 of 20 questions correctly, do I pass? ...............................................................................................yes, I get 75

22. One bag of corn will plant 3 acres, how many bags for 90 acres?............................30

23. If I pay my gas bill on time I get 10% off. My bill is $29.00. How much do I get off?...................................................................................................................$2.90

24. Of 1000 people, 35% smoke. How many smoke?...................................................350

# MATH
## CREATED BY GLENN SEYMOUR

1. A farmer picks 10 acres of corn in one hour.  How long will it take to pick 80 acres?_____

2. A man has 40 hogs, sells 25%. How many does he have left?_____

3. A tank holds 200 gallon. If it is 1/4 full how many gallons does it have in it? _____

4. If a cow gives 5 gallon of milk a day, how much does she give in a week? _____

5. If you feed one horse 3 ears of corn, how many ears do you need for 15 horses?_____

6. If you spend $20.00 playing a slot machine and win $7.00, how much did you lose? _____
   _____

7. If you bought a suit for $120.00, a second one was 1/2 price, how much would two suits cost you?_____

8. I purchased 70 eggs, fell down and broke half of them. How many did I have left?_____

9. A 2 1/2 gallon bucket of water leaks 1/2 gallon per hour. How long will it take to empty the bucket? _____

10. When I planted beans 2 out of 3 came up. What percentage that I planted grew?_____

11. Candy bars are 4 for 20 cents. If I buy 5 candy bars how much do I owe? _____

12. My car gets 25 miles on a gallon of gas. If I go 200 miles how many gallons of gas will I need? _____

13. If 4 cows eat one bale of hay, how many bales will 12 cows eat? _____

14. If I worked 2 1/2 hours at $5.00 per hour, how much money did I make? _____

15. Pick your own berries are 25 cents a quart. We pick 40 cents worth of berries. How much difference? _____

16. I purchase a small chain at 8 cents per foot.  How much will I pay for 4 feet?  _____

17. If asparagus grew 4 inches a day, how tall is it in one week? _____

18. A balloon floats along at 12 miles per hour, how long will it take the balloon to go 60 miles? _____

19. A pump pumps 25 gallon of water in a minute.  How much will it pump in 5 minutes? _____

20. I needed change for 50 cents. I wanted one quarter, one dime, and one nickel. How much more change do I have coming?_____

21. I leave for home at 12:30. It takes 3 1/2 hours for me to get home. What time will I arrive?

22. I pay my utilities quarterly. How many times a year do I pay?_____

23. My rent is $400.00. If I pay late I must add 5%. When I am late how much must I pay? ___

24. Cookies are 2 for 25 cents. How much for 8 cookies? _____

25. Cookies are 2 for 25 cents. How much for one dozen? _____

# MATH
## CREATED BY GLENN SEYMOUR

1. A farmer picks 10 acres of corn in one hour. How long will it take to pick 80 acres? ...8 hours

2. A man has 40 hogs, sells 25%. How many does he have left?........................................ 30 hogs

3. A tank holds 200 gallon. If it is 1/4 full how many gallons does it have in it?....................50 gallon

4. If a cow gives 5 gallon of milk a day, how much does she give in a week? ...............35 gallon

5. If you feed one horse 3 ears of corn, how many ears do you need for 15 horses?..........45 ears

6. If you spend $20.00 playing a slot machine and win $7.00, how much did you lose?..... $13.00

7. If you bought a suit for $120.00, a second one was 1/2 price, how much would two suits cost you? .....................................................................................................................$180.00

8. I purchased 70 eggs, fell down and broke half of them. How many did I have left?.......35 eggs

9. A 2 1/2 gallon bucket of water leaks 1/2 gallon per hour. How long will it take to empty the bucket? ................................................................................................................5 hours

10. When I planted beans 2 out of 3 came up. What percentage that I planted grew? .........2/3%

11. Candy bars are 4 for 20 cents. If I buy 5 candy bars how much do I owe?......................... 25¢

12. My car gets 25 miles on a gallon of gas. If I go 200 miles how many gallons of gas will I need? ........................................................................................................................8 gallon

13. If 4 cows eat one bale of hay, how many bales will 12 cows eat? ...................................3 bales

14. If I worked 2 1/2 hours at $5.00 per hour, how much money did I make?.................... $12.50

15. Pick your own berries are 25 cents a quart. We pick 40 cents worth of berries. How much difference? .................................................................................................................. 15¢

16. I purchase a small chain at 8 cents per foot. How much will I pay for 4 feet? ................ 32¢

17. If asparagus grew 4 inches a day, how tall is it in one week?...................................... 28 inches

18. A balloon floats along at 12 miles per hour, how long will it take the balloon to go 60 miles? .......................................................................................................................5 hours

19. A pump pumps 25 gallon of water in a minute. How much will it pump in 5 minutes?. 125 gal.

20. I needed change for 50 cents. I wanted one quarter, one dime, and one nickel. How much more change do I have coming?................................................................................... 10¢

21. I leave for home at 12:30. It takes 3 1/2 hours for me to get home. What time will I arrive?... 4:00

22. I pay my utilities quarterly. How many times a year do I pay? .................................................4

23. My rent is $400.00. If I pay late I must ad 5%. When I am late how much must I pay? ... $420.00

24. Cookies are 2 for 25 cents. How much for 8 cookies?.................................................... $1.00

25. Cookies are 2 for 25 cents. How much for one dozen?.................................................... $1.50

# MATH
## CREATED BY GLENN SEYMOUR

1.  Distance from one end of the hall to another is?_____

2.  Distance from side to side is? _____

3.  Distance from floor to ceiling is. _____

4.  What is a square?_____

5.  How many degrees in a right angle? _____

6.  How many degrees with four angles of a square? _____

7.  Vertical line is? _____

8.  Parallel line is?_____

9.  Describe a circle _____

10. The distance around a circle is? _____

11. Distance across the widest point is? _____

12. One half the diameter is? _____

13. Degrees in a circle is? _____

14. What is a block or dice called? _____

15. How many sides to a block or cube? _____

16. What is the amount a tank holds? _____

17. To find the circumference of a circle _____

18. What is a vertical line? _____

# MATH
## CREATED BY GLENN SEYMOUR

1.  Distance from one end of the hall to another is? ................................................. length

2.  Distance from side to side is? ................................................................................ width

3.  Distance from floor to ceiling is. ......................................................................... height

4.  What is a square? .......................................................... figure with four sides of equal length

5.  How many degrees in a right angle? ............................................................................. 90

6.  How many degrees with four angles of a square? ..................................................... 360

7.  Vertical line is? ................................................................................................. up and down

8.  Parallel line is? ...................... two or more lines that remain the same distance apart

9.  Describe a circle ............................................................................... round loop or hoop

10. The distance around a circle is? ........................................................ circumference

11. Distance across the widest point is? ....................................................... diameter

12. One half the diameter is? ............................................................................... radius

13. Degrees in a circle is? ....................................................................................... 360

14. What is a block or dice called? ...................................................................... cube

15. How many sides to a block or cube? ................................................................... 6

16. What is the amount a tank holds? ..................................... volume - quarts - barrels

17. To find the circumference of a circle ........................................... diameter times pi

18. What is a vertical line? ........................................................................ level length wise

# MISC.

# TALES & NURSERY RHYMES
## CREATED BY GLENN SEYMOUR

1.  Rub a Dub, how many men in a tub?_____

2.  To market to market to buy?_____

3.  What three things did Old King Cole call for?_____

4.  Tom Thumb the Pipers Son stole a_____

5.  What happened to the pig?_____

6.  What happened to Tom?_____

7.  Where was Rock A Bye Baby?_____

8.  What if the brough breaks?_____

9.  What question is asked in BaBaBlack Sheep?_____

10. How much wool?_____

11. Who were the wool for?_____

12. What happened to Chicken Little?_____

13. What did she say?_____

14. Where did Mary's Little Lamb go?_____

15. What was Humpty Dumpty?_____

16. What happened to him?_____

17. What was he sitting on?_____

18. Who were the Three Blind Mice running after?_____

19. What did she do?_____

20. What did Jack Be Nimble jump over?_____

21. Where was Little Red Riding Hood going and why?_____

22. Who was there?_____

23. What three questions did she ask the wolf?_____

24. Where had Pussy Cat been?_____

25. What did she do there?_____

# TALES & NURSERY RHYMES
## CREATED BY GLENN SEYMOUR

1. Rub a dub how many men in at tub? ...................................................................3

2. To market to market to buy ....................................................................a fat pig

3. What three things did Old King Cole call for?....................pipe, bowl, fiddlers three

4. Tom Thumb the Pipers son stole a.............................................................pig

5. What happened to the pig? ......................................got loose, caught a goose

6. What happened to Tom? ...................................... got caught, put in calaboose

7. Where was Rock A Bye Baby? ........................................................ in the tree top

8. What if the bough breaks? ........ cradle will fall, down will come baby, cradle and all

9. What question is asked in BaBaBlack Sheep?...................................have you any wool

10. How much wool?............................................................................ three bags full

11. Who were the wool for?........................ master, dame. Little boy that lives in the lane

12. What happened to Chicken Little? ................................................acorn fell on her head

13. What did she say?............................................. the sky is falling, come with me

14. Where did Mary's Little Lamb go? ........................................................to school one day

15. What was Humpty Dumpty? ...................................................................... egg

16. What happened to him? ...................................................... he had  a great fall

17. What was he sitting on?...........................................................................wall

18. Who were the Three Blind Mice running after?...............................the farmers wife

19. What did she do?.................................................cut off their tails with a butchers knife

20. What did Jack be Nimble jump over?...............................................................candlestick

21. Where was little Red Riding Hood going and why?........ to Grandma's house to take cookies

22. Who was there? ...................................................................................... wolf

23. What three questions did she ask the wolf?...... what big ears, big eyes, big teeth you have

24. Where had Pussy Cat been?............................................... to London to see the Queen

25. What did she do there?................................frighten the mouse from under her chair

# COLORS
## CREATED BY GLENN SEYMOUR

### SEVEN WAYS TO CHANGE COLORS

1. ......................................................................................................................................

2. ......................................................................................................................................

3. ......................................................................................................................................

4. ......................................................................................................................................

5. ......................................................................................................................................

6. ......................................................................................................................................

7. ......................................................................................................................................

### PERSONS OR FAMILIES IN COLOR

1. ......................................................................................................................................

2. ......................................................................................................................................

3. ......................................................................................................................................

4. ......................................................................................................................................

5. ......................................................................................................................................

6. ......................................................................................................................................

7. ......................................................................................................................................

8. ......................................................................................................................................

9. ......................................................................................................................................

10. ......................................................................................................................................

11. ......................................................................................................................................

12. ......................................................................................................................................

# COLORS
CREATED BY GLENN SEYMOUR

## SEVEN WAYS TO CHANGE COLORS

1. ................................................................................................DYE
2. ............................................................................................SHADE
3. ..............................................................................................TINT
4. ............................................................................................PAINT
5. ............................................................................................STAIN
6. .............................................................................................FADE
7. ..........................................................................................BLEACH

## PERSONS OR FAMILIES IN COLOR

1. ...........................................................................................WHITE
2. ...........................................................................................BLACK
3. ..........................................................................................BROWN
4. ...........................................................................................GREEN
5. .............................................................................................GRAY
6. .............................................................................................RUBY
7. ..........................................................................................LEMON
8. .............................................................................................ROSE
9. .............................................................................................KELLY
10. ........................................................................................AMBER
11. ......................................................................................SCARLET
12. ...........................................................................................RUST

# "TEASERS"
## CREATED BY GLENN SEYMOUR

1.  What has uppers and lowers but no teeth?_____

2.  What has ears but can't hear?_____

3.  What has eyes but can't see?_____

4.  What has teeth but can't bite?_____

5.  What has keys that will not open a lock?_____

6.  What besides the Army has a Colonel (kernel)?_____

7.  What has a mouth but can't eat?_____

8.  What has a back that won't bend?_____

9.  What has 5 fingers but no feeling?_____

10. What has no legs but runs?_____

11. What has a tongue but can't taste_____

12. What goes around & around but stays in the same place?_____

13. Why never tell secrets in a cornfield?_____

14. What goes up & down but stays in place?_____

15. Name a bad tempered apple._____

16. What part of hairstyle is a loud sound?_____

17. Name a yummy apple._____

18. What orange bears the name of the body?_____

19. How many sides to a circle?_____

# "TEASERS"
## CREATED BY GLENN SEYMOUR

1.  What has uppers and lowers but no teeth? ........................................ bunk beds
2.  What has ears but can't hear? ........................................................ corn
3.  What has eyes but can't see? ......................................................... potato
4.  What has teeth but can't bite? ...................................................... comb
5.  What has keys that won't open a lock? .......................................... piano
6.  What besides the Army has a Colonel (kernel)? ........................... ear of corn
7.  What has a mouth but can't eat? .................................................... river
8.  What has a back that won't bend? ................................................. chair
9.  What has 5 fingers but no feeling? ................................................ glove
10. What has no legs but runs? ........................................................... river
11. What has a tongue but can't taste? ............................................... shoe
12. What goes around & around but stays in place? .......................... clock
13. Why never tell secrets in a cornfield? ........................ because of all the ears
14. What goes up & down but stays in place? ................................... pump handle
15. Name a bad tempered apple ......................................................... crab
16. What part of hairstyle is a loud sound ........................................ bangs
17. Name a yummy apple ................................................................... delicious
18. What orange bears the name of a body? ..................................... navel
19. How many sides to a circle? ........................................ 2 inside & outside

# SUPERSTITIOUS SAYINGS
## CREATED BY GLENN SEYMOUR

1. One who gets in on none of the good things or times is_____

2. A bad penny always_____

3. Eat cabbage on New Years Day for a _____

4. Spilling salt is_____

5. Bad luck to give a knife unless they_____

6. Bird flies against a window is_____

7. Drop dish cloth on the floor means_____

8. Drop a fork means_____

9. Raising umbrella in the house means_____

10. Sweep dirt out the door_____

11. Leave, return for something is_____

12. Enter by one door, leave by another door_____

13. Find a coin heads up is_____

14. Break a mirror is_____

15. Find a four leaf clover is_____

16. Rain Easter Sunday and it will_____

17. Groundhog sees his shadow means_____

18. Rain on Monday and it will_____

19. Whirlwind in fields is a_____

20. Black or dark wollyworms mean_____

21. Light wollyworms mean_____

22. Persimmon seeds shape of spoon or shovel_____

23. A body will not rust but _____

24. Snow flurries, rain & wind in May_____

25. Sing before breakfast_____

26. Itchy palm_____

# SUPERSTITIOUS SAYINGS
## CREATED BY GLENN SEYMOUR

1.  One who gets in on none of the good things or times is.......a day late and a dollar short

2.  A bad penny always ............................................................................... returns

3.  Eat cabbage on News Years Day for a .........................................................good year

4.  Spilling salt is ...............................................................................................bad luck

5.  Bad luck to give a knife unless they ........................................give you a coin

6.  Bird flies against a window is.....................................................sign of a death

7.  Drop dish cloth on floor means....................................someone unclean is coming

8.  Drop a fork means................................. company coming from direction tines point

9.  Raising umbrella in the house means............................................... bad luck

10. Sweep dirt out the door .........................................sweep away your fortune

11. Leave, return for something is..................................................... bad luck

12. Enter by one door, leave by another door ......................................company is coming

13. Find a coin heads up ...................................................................good luck

14. Break a mirror is............................................................... 7 years bad luck

15. Find a four leaf clover is .............................................................good luck

16. Rain Easter Sunday and it will................................. rain the next seven Sundays

17. Groundhog sees his shadow means ........................................ six more weeks Winter

18. Rain on Monday and it will....................................... rain three days that week

19. Whirlwind in fields is a ................................................ sign of dry weather

20. Black or dark wollyworms means .......................................................hard Winter.

21. Light wollyworms means ..................................................... mild Winter

22. Persimmon seeds shape of spoon or shovel.............................................lots of snow

23. A body will not rust out but................................................. wear out

24. Snow flurries, rain & wind in May......................................blackberry Winter

25. Sing before breakfast...............................................................cry before supper

26. Itchy palm................................................................. going to get money

124

# SUPERSTITIOUS SAYINGS
## CREATED BY GLENN SEYMOUR

1.  Do unto others as you_____

2.  Never put off until tomorrow_____

3.  Don't believe anything you hear and only_____

4.  Absence makes the heart_____

5.  When the going gets tough_____

6.  If at first you don't succeed_____

7.  Two sure things in life are_____

8.  An apple a day_____

9.  Judge not_____

10. People in glass houses_____

11. The grass is always greener_____

12. Necessity is the father of_____

13. He who hesitates_____

14. Don't let anyone pull_____

15. Don't let someone sell you_____

16. If a deal sounds too good to be true_____

17. You seldom get something_____

18. All that glitters_____

19. Charge it to the dust and_____

20. It goes in one ear and_____

21. Early to bed and early to rise_____

# SUPERSTITIOUS SAYINGS
## CREATED BY GLENN SEYMOUR

1. Do unto others as you................................................................would have them do unto you

2. Never put off until tomorrow .....................................................what you can do today

3. Don't believe anything you hear and only....................................half of what you see

4. Absence makes the heart.............................................................grow fonder

5. When the going gets tough ..........................................................the tough get going

6. If at first you don't succeed.........................................................try, try again

7. Two sure things in life are ..........................................................death - taxes

8. An apple a day............................................................................keeps the doctor away

9. Judge not....................................................................................lest you be judged

10. People in glass houses...............................................................should never throw stones

11. The grass is always greener.........................................................on the other side of the street

12. Necessity is the father of............................................................invention

13. He who hesitates........................................................................fails

14. Don't let anyone pull..................................................................the wool over your eyes

15. Don't let someone sell you...........................................................a pig in a poke

16. If a deal sounds too good to be true ............................................the chances are it is

17. You seldom get something ..........................................................for nothing

18. All that glitters ..........................................................................is not gold

19. Charge it to the dust and ............................................................let the rain settle it

20. It goes in one ear and.................................................................and out the other

21. Early to bed and early to rise .......................................makes a man healthy, wealthy and wise

# PEOPLE, RADIO & TV

# WELL KNOWS NAMES
## CREATED BY GLENN SEYMOUR

1. Tony _____

2. Nathan _____

3. Orson _____

4. John Wilkes _____

5. Fanny _____

6. Tennessee Ernie _____

7. Walter _____

8. Buddy _____

9. Marlon _____

10. Buster _____

11. Oprah _____

12. Walt _____

13. Nat King _____

14. Harpo _____

15. Carney _____

16. Lon _____

17. Gleason _____

18. Walter _____

19. Charlton _____

20. Burl _____

21. Irvin _____

22. John Quincy _____

23. Marilyn _____

24. Pat - Daniel _____

25. Johnny _____

26. Lyndon Baines _____

27. Jacqueline Kennedy _____

28. Eleanor (wife) _____

29. Lincoln (wife) _____

30. Richard _____

31. Ronald _____

32. Gerald Ford (wife) _____

33. Foxx _____

34. Rev. Billy _____

35. Chet _____

36. Elizabeth _____

# WELL KNOWN NAMES
CREATED BY GLENN SEYMOUR

1. Tony ............................. Orlando
2. Nathan ..........................Hale
3. Orson .......................... Wells
4. John Wilkes................... Boothe
5. Fanny .........................Brice
6. Tennessee Ernie.................Ford
7. Walter ...........................Brennen
8. Buddy.............................Epson
9. Marlon ..........................Brando
10. Buster........................... Keaton
11. Oprah.......................... Winfrey
12. Walt.............................Disney
13. Nat King .............................Cole
14. Harpo............................. Marx
15. Carney ................................Art
16. Lon ............................. Chaney
17. Gleason...........................Jackie
18. Walter ........................ Winchell
19. Charlton ........................ Heston
20. Burl .......................................Ives
21. Irving ............................... Berlin
22. John Quincy...................Adams
23. Marilyn .......................Monroe
24. Pat - Daniel .................... Boone
25. Johnny ...............Carson - Cash
26. Lyndon Baines............. Johnson
27. Jacqueline Kennedy .......Onasis
28. Eleanor (wife) ...........Roosevelt
29. Lincoln (wife) ........ Mary Todd
30. Richard ...........................Nixon
31. Ronald ...........................Regean
32. Gerald Ford (wife) ...........Betty
33. Foxx................................Redd
34. Rev. Billy...................... Graham
35. Chet................................ Atkins
36. Elizabeth..........................Taylor

# WHO, WHAT SHOW
CREATED BY GLENN SEYMOUR

1. Who says "Here's Johnny?"_____

2. Who says "What is the secret word?"_____

3. Who sings "Singing In The Rain?"_____

4. Who is known as "Old Blue Eyes?"_____

5. Who is known as "Ski Nose?"_____

6. Who said "Howdy I'm So Proud To Be Here?"_____

7. Who is "Uncle Milty?"_____

8. Who said "Goodnight Gracie?"_____

9. Who was the "Galloping Ghost?"_____

10. Who was nicknamed "Dino?"_____

11. Who was the "Greatest?"_____

12. Who is the "Man in Black?"_____

13. Who is the "Coal Miners Daughter?"_____

14. Who is the "Storyteller?"_____

15. Who is the "Rhinestone Cowboy?"_____

16. Who said "Kids Say The Dandiest Things?"_____

17. Who says "What's My Line?"_____

18. Who plays the part of a drunk?_____

19. Who stutters?_____

20. Who MC's The Muscular Dystopia Show?_____

21. Who is "I Love Lucy?"_____

22. Whose Husband was called Fang?_____

23. Who said "We Will Return?"_____

24. Who is "Wilt the Stilt?"_____

25. Who is "Tater?"_____

# WHO - WHAT SHOW?
## CREATED BY GLENN SEYMOUR

1. Who says "Here's Johnny?" .................................................................. Ed McMahon

2. Who says "What is the secret word?" ................................. Groucho Marx

3. Who sings "Singing in the Rain?" ........................................... Gene Kelly

4. Who is known as "Old Blue Eyes?" ..................................... Frank Sinatra

5. Who is known as "Ski Nose?" .................................................... Bob Hope

6. Who said "Howdy I'm so Proud to be here?" ..................... Minnie Pearl

7. Who is Uncle Milty? .................................................................. Milton Berle

8. Who said "Goodnight Gracie?" ............................................. George Burns

9. Who was the "Galloping Ghost?" ........................................... Red Grange

10. Who was nicknamed "Dino?" ................................................. Dean Martin

11. Who was the "Greatest?" ..................................................... Muhammad Ali

12. Who was the "Man in Black?" .................................................. Johnny Cash

13. Who is the "Coal Miners Daughter?" .................................... Loretta Lynn

14. Who is the "Storyteller?" ......................................................... Tom T. Hall

15. Who is the "Rhinestone Cowboy?" ................................... Glenn Campbell

16. Who said "Kids Say The Darndest Things?" ...................... Art Linkletter

17. Who says "What's My Line?" .................................................. Gary Moore

18. Who plays the part of a drunk? .......................................... Foster Brooks

19. Who stutters? ............................................................................. Mel Tellis

20. Who MC's the Muscular Dystrophy Show? .......................... Jerry Lewis

21. Who is "I Love Lucy?" ............................................................ Lucille Ball

22. Whose Husband was called Fang? ...................................... Phyllis Diller

23. Who said "We Shall Return?" .......................... General Douglas McArthur

24. Who is "Wilt the Stilt?" ................................................. Wilt Chamberlain

25. Who is "Tater?" .............................................. Little Jimmy Dickens

# WELL KNOWN NAMES
CREATED BY GLENN SEYMOUR

1.  David &_____

2.  Amos &_____

3.  Lum &_____

4.  Jack &_____

5.  Bob Hope &_____

6.  Fibber McGee &_____

7.  Dean Martin &_____

8.  Mutt &_____

9.  Tom &_____

10. Lewis &_____

11. Adam &_____

12. Sonny &_____

13. Roy Rogers &_____

14. Bert &_____

15. Huntley &_____

16. Pat &_____

17. Porky &_____

18. Carson &_____

19. Tarzan &_____

20. Rogers &_____

21. Jackie Gleason &_____

22. Romeo &_____

23. Long Ranger &_____

24. Johnson &_____

25. Ozzie &_____

26. Homer &_____

27. Lula Belle &_____

28. Frick &_____

29. Popeye &_____

30. Burns &_____

31. Sherri Lewis &_____

32. Sears &_____

33. Red Skelton &_____

34. Lucille Ball &_____

35. Jimmy Durante &_____

36. Hans &_____

# WELL KNOWN NAMES
## CREATED BY GLENN SEYMOUR

1. David & ..................................... Goliath
2. Amos & .....................................Andy
3. Lum & ..................................... Abner
4. Jack & .....................................Jill
5. Bob Hope & ...................Bing Crosby
6. Fibber Magee & ....................... Molly
7. Dean Martin & .................Jerry Lewis
8. Mutt & .....................................Jeff
9. Tom & .....................................Jerry
10. Lewis & .....................................Clark
11. Adam & ..................................... Eve
12. Sonny & .....................................Cher
13. Roy Rogers & ...................Dale Evans
14. Bert & .....................................Ernie
15. Huntley & ......................... Brinkley
16. Pat & ..................................... Mike
17. Porky .....................................Bess
18. Carson & ...........................McMahon
19. Tarzan & .....................................Jane
20. Rogers & ..................... Hammerstein
21. Jackie Gleason & .............Art Carney
22. Romeo & ..................................... Juliet
23. Lone Ranger & ......................... Tonto
24. Johnson & ..............................Johnson
25. Ozzie & .....................................Harriet
26. Homer & .....................................Jethro
27. Lula Belle & ..............................Scotty
28. Frick & .....................................Frack
29. Popeye & ............................. Olive Oil
30. Burns & .....................................Allen
31. Sherri Lewis & .................Lamb Chop
32. Sears & .....................................Roebuck
33. Red Skelton & ..................................... Clem Kadiddle Hopper
34. Lucille Ball & ...................Desi Arnaz
35. Jimmy Durante & ...... Mrs. Calabash
36. Hans & .....................................Gretel

# FAMOUS NAMES 1
CREATED BY GLENN SEYMOUR

1. Gardner _____

2. Garth _____

3. Gabby _____

4. Burns _____

5. Boxcar _____

6. Alfred _____

7. Audrey _____

8. Buddy _____

9. Campbell _____

10. Coolidge _____

11. Carter _____

12. Cass _____

13. Cosby _____

14. Sally _____

15. Imogene _____

16. Crosby _____

17. J. P. _____

18. Andrew _____

19. Joan _____

20. Jerry _____

21. Durante _____

22. Jolson _____

23. Jordan _____

24. Booth _____

25. John Quincy _____

26. John Wilkes _____

27. Buster _____

28. Lois _____

29. Landers _____

30. Murray _____

31. Gish _____

32. Mamie _____

33. McMahan _____

34. Rather _____

35. Griffin _____

36. Quayle _____

# FAMOUS NAMES 1
## CREATED BY GLENN SEYMOUR

1. Gardner ..................................... Ava
2. Garth ..................................... Brooks
3. Gabby ..................................... Hayes
4. Burns ..................................... George
5. Boxcar ..................................... Willie
6. Alfred ..................................... Hitchcock
7. Audrey ..................................... Meadows
8. Buddy ..................................... Hackett
9. Campbell ..................................... Bill
10. Coolidge ..................................... Calvin
11. Carter ..................................... Jimmy
12. Cass ..................................... Peggy
13. Cosby ..................................... Bob
14. Sally ..................................... Rand
15. Imogene ..................................... Coca
16. Crosby ..................................... Bing
17. J. P. ..................................... Morgan
18. Andrew ..................................... Jackson
19. Joan ..................................... Crawford
20. Jerry ..................................... Lewis
21. Durante ..................................... Jimmy
22. Jolson ..................................... Al
23. Jordan ..................................... Michael
24. Booth ..................................... Shirley
25. John Quincy ..................................... Adams
26. John Wilkes ..................................... Booth
27. Buster ..................................... Keaton
28. Lois ..................................... Lane
29. Landers ..................................... Ann - Abby
30. Murray ..................................... Anne
31. Gish ..................................... Lillian
32. Mamie ..................................... Eisenhower
33. McMahan ..................................... Ed
34. Rather ..................................... Dan
35. Griffin ..................................... Merv
36. Quayle ..................................... Dan

136

# FAMOUS NAMES 2
CREATED BY GLENN SEYMOUR

1. Jonas Salk_____

2. Henry Ford_____

3. Ben Franklin_____

4. Alexander Graham Bell_____

5. Eli Whitney_____

6. Sir Isaac Newton_____

7. Robert J. Fulton_____

8. Lous Pasteur_____

9. Ripley_____

10. McCormick_____

11. Norman Rockwell_____

12. Billy Graham_____

13. Walter Cronkite_____

14. Danny Thomas_____

15. Helen Keller_____

16. Evil Knevil_____

17. Kreston_____

18. Daniel Webster_____

19. Elisha Otis_____

20. Dr. Benjamin Spock_____

21. Amelia Earhart_____

22. Emmet Kelley_____

23. Betsy Ross_____

24. Francis Scott Key_____

25. Boots Randolph_____

26. John Wilkes Booth_____

# FAMOUS NAMES 2
## CREATED BY GLENN SEYMOUR

1.  Jonas Salk ....................................................................................... polio Vaccine
2.  Henry Ford ....................................................................................... model T
3.  Ben Franklin ..................................................................................... electricity
4.  Alexander Graham Bell .................................................................... telephone
5.  Eli Whitney ...................................................................................... cotton gin
6.  Sir Isaac Newton .............................................................................. gravity
7.  Robert J. Fulton ............................................................................... steamboat
8.  Lous Pasteur .................................................................................... pasteurizing
9.  Ripley ............................................................................................... believe or not
10. McCormick ...................................................................................... spices / tractor
11. Norman Rockwell ........................................................................... Saturday Evening Post
12. Billy Graham .................................................................................... evangelist
13. Walter Cronkite ............................................................................... newsman
14. Danny Thomas ................................................................................ comedian
15. Helen Keller .................................................................................... blind - published a book
16. Evil Knevil ....................................................................................... daredevil
17. Kreston ............................................................................................ mindreader
18. Daniel Webster ................................................................................ dictionary
19. Elisha Otis ....................................................................................... elevator
20. Dr. Benjamin Spock ........................................................................ baby doctor
21. Amelia Earhart ................................................................................ aviator
22. Emmet Kelly .................................................................................... clown
23. Betsy Ross ....................................................................................... American flag
24. Francis Scott Key ............................................................................ wrote Star Bungled Banner
25. Boots Randolph ............................................................................... trumpet player
26. John Wilkes Booth .......................................................................... assassinated Abe Lincoln

# FAMOUS NAMES 3
## CREATED BY GLENN SEYMOUR

1. Rivers _____

2. Mathis _____

3. Farrow _____

4. Reddy _____

5. Diller _____

6. Rogers _____

7. O'Brien _____

8. Page _____

9. Parks _____

10. VanDyke _____

11. Travis _____

12. Thomas _____

13. Sophie _____

14. Tex _____

15. Sullivan _____

16. Goldwater _____

17. Ozzie & _____

18. Mineo _____

19. Monty _____

20. Mudd _____

21. Edward R. _____

22. Reese _____

23. Shore _____

24. Zackary _____

25. Marx _____

26. Zane _____

27. Wonder _____

28. Welk _____

29. Reynolds _____

30. Bombeck _____

31. Edgar Allan _____

32. Ulysses S. _____

33. Booker T. _____

34. Warren G. _____

35. Grover _____

36. Sir Isaac _____

# FAMOUS NAMES 3
## CREATED BY GLENN SEYMOUR

1. Rivers ................................ Joan
2. Mathis ............................. Johnny
3. Farrow ............................... Mia
4. Reddy ............................... Helen
5. Diller .............................. Phyllis
6. Rogers ................. Will - Dale - Roy
7. O'Brien ............................. Pat
8. Page ............................... Patti
9. Park ............................... Bert
10. VanDyke .................. Dick - Jerry
11. Travis .............................. Randy
12. Thomas ............................ Danny
13. Sophie ............................ Tucker
14. Tex ................................ Ritter
15. Sullivan ............................. Ed
16. Goldwater ........................ Barry
17. Ozzie & .......................... Harriet
18. Mineo ............................... Sal

19. Monty ............................. Hall
20. Mudd ............................. Roger
21. Edward R ...................... Murrow
22. Reese .............................. Della
23. Shore ............................. Dinah
24. Zackary ........................... Taylor
25. Marx ........................... Grouxho
26. Zane .............................. Gray
27. Wonder .......................... Stevie
28. Welk ........................... Lawrence
29. Reynolds ......................... Debbie
30. Bombeck .......................... Erma
31. Edgar Allen ........................ Poe
32. Ulysses S .......................... Grant
33. Booker T ................... Washington
34. Warren G ....................... Harding
35. Grover ......................... Cleveland
36. Sir Isaac ........................ Newton

# FAMOUS NAMES 4
## CREATED BY GLENN SEYMOUR

1. Ben ..........................................................................................................

2. Henry ........................................................................................................

3. Harry S. ....................................................................................................

4. Nathan .......................................................................................................

5. Nixon .........................................................................................................

6. Orson .........................................................................................................

7. Theodore....................................................................................................

8. Sandberg....................................................................................................

9. Rutherford B. ............................................................................................

10. Cole ..........................................................................................................

11. Tennessee...................................................................................................

12. Colon .........................................................................................................

13. Douglas......................................................................................................

14. Revere .......................................................................................................

15. Adolph .......................................................................................................

16. Presley........................................................................................................

17. Susan B. .....................................................................................................

18. Jonas ..........................................................................................................

19. Rockwell ....................................................................................................

20. Doris...........................................................................................................

21. Amelia ........................................................................................................

22. Autry ..........................................................................................................

23. Babe............................................................................................................

24. Abegale ......................................................................................................

# FAMOUS NAMES 4
## CREATED BY GLENN SEYMOUR

1. Ben ........................................................................................................... Franklin

2. Henry ........................................................................................................... Ford

3. Harry S ...................................................................................................... Truman

4. Nathan .......................................................................................................... Hale

5. Nixon ....................................................................................................... Richard

6. Orson ........................................................................................................... Wells

7. Theodore ................................................................................................ Roosevelt

8. Sandberg ........................................................................................................ Carl

9. Rutherford B ............................................................................................... Hayes

10. Cole ...................................................................................................... Nat King

11. Tennessee ........................................................................................... Ernie Ford

12. Colon ......................................................................................................... Powell

13. Douglas ................................................................................................ McArthur

14. Revere ............................................................................................................ Paul

15. Adolph ........................................................................................................ Hitler

16. Presley ........................................................................................................... Elvis

17. Susan B ..................................................................................................... Anthony

18. Jonas ............................................................................................................. Saul

19. Rockwell ................................................................................................... Norman

20. Doris .............................................................................................................. Day

21. Amelia ....................................................................................................... Earhart

22. Autry ............................................................................................................ Gene

23. Babe ............................................................................................................. Ruth

24. Abigail .................................................................................................... Van Buren

# RADIO & TV SHOWS
### CREATED BY GLENN SEYMOUR

1. The Jack _____ Show

2. The Doris _____ Show

3. The Dinah_____ Show

4. The Jerry_____ Show

5. The Groucho _____ Show

6. The Julia _____ Show

7. The Dick_____ Show

8. The Jackie _____ Show

9. The Bob _____ Show

10. The Ed _____ Show

11. The Mary Tyler_____ Show

12. The Johnny _____ Show

13. The Red _____ Show

14. The Redd _____ Show

15. The Merv _____ Show

16. The Ralph_____ Show

17. The George_____ Show

18. The David_____ Show

19. The Statler _____ Show

20. The John _____ Show

21. The Donna _____ Show

22. The Johnny _____ Show

23. The Jimmy _____ Show

24. The Porter_____ Show

25. The Oprah _____ Show

26. The Edgar _____ Show

27. The Marlin _____ Show

28. The Mel_____ Show

29. The Alfred _____ Show

30. The Will _____ Show

31. The Burns & _____ Show

32. The Bob _____ Show

33. Lulla Belle &_____ Show

34. Regis & _____ Show

# RADIO & TV SHOWS
## CREATED BY GLENN SEYMOUR

1.  The Jack _____Paar_____ Show
2.  The Doris _____Day_____ Show
3.  The Dinah _____Shore_____ Show
4.  The Jerry _____Lewis_____ Show
5.  The Groucho _Marx_____ Show
6.  The Julia _____Childs_____ Show
7.  The Dick _____Van Dyke_____ Show
8.  The Jackie _____Gleason_____ Show
9.  The Bob _____Hope_____ Show
10. The Ed _____Sullivan_____ Show
11. The Mary Tyler _Moore_____ Show
12. The Johnny _____Carson_____ Show
13. The Red _____Skelton_____ Show
14. The Redd _____Foxx_____ Show
15. The Merv _____Griffin_____ Show
16. The Ralph _____Emery_____ Show
17. The George _____Goble_____ Show

18. The David _____Letterman_____ Show
19. The Statler _____Brothers_____ Show
20. The John _____Denver_____ Show
21. The Donna _____Reed_____ Show
22. The Johnny _____Cash_____ Show
23. The Jimmy _____Dean_____ Show
24. The Porter _____Wagoner_____ Show
25. The Oprah _____Winfrey_____ Show
26. The Edgar _____Bergen_____ Show
27. The Marlin _____Perkins_____ Show
28. The Mel _____Tullis_____ Show
29. The Alfred _____Hitchcock_____ Show
30. The Will _____Rogers_____ Show
31. The Burns & _Allen_____ Show
32. The Bob _____Newhart_____ Show
33. Lulla Belle & _Scotty_____ Show
34. Regis & _____Cathy Lee_____ Show

# RADIO & TV SHOWS - PAST & PRESENT
### CREATED BY GLENN SEYMOUR

1. All in the_____

2. The Three _____

3. Petty Coat_____

4. My Three _____

5. The Lone_____

6. This Old _____

7. This is Your_____

8. Murder She_____

9. Father Knows _____

10. Little House on the_____

11. As The World _____

12. Grand Ole_____

13. Name That _____

14. Leave it to _____

15. The Days of Our _____

16. The Guiding _____

17. Lets Make A _____

18. Sixty _____

19. The Match _____

20. I Love _____

21. You Bet Your_____

22. The Young and the _____

23. Truth or _____

24. Candid _____

25. The Price is_____

26. I've Got A _____

27. Wheel of_____

28. Green _____

29. My Mother the _____

30. Kids Say The_____

31. The Hee Haw _____

32. The Beverly_____

33. Gilligan's_____

34. Beat the_____

35. Sesame _____

36. WLS _____

# RADIO & TV SHOWS PAST & PRESENT
## CREATED BY GLENN SEYMOUR

1. All In The .................................Family
2. The Three ............................ Stooges
3. Petty Coat ...........................Junction
4. My Three .............................. Sons
5. The Lone .................................Ranger
6. This Old.................................. House
7. This is Your .................................Life
8. Murder She ...............................Wrote
9. Father Knows ............................ Best
10. Little House On The ..............Prairie
11. As The World...........................Turns
12. Grand Ole ................................. Opry
13. Name That .................................Tune
14. Leave It To...............................Beaver
15. The Days of Our........................Lives
16. The Guiding............................. Light
17. Let Make A ............................ Deal
18. Sixty .......................................... Minutes

19. The Match .................................Game
20. I Love.........................................Lucy
21. You Bet Your.................................Life
22. The Young and The..............Restless
23. Truth or ..................... Consequences
24. Candid.....................................Camera
25. The Price Is ................................Right
26. I've Got A .................................Secret
27. Wheel Of................................Fortune
28. Green......................................... Acres
29. My Mother The ............................Car
30. Kids Say The .............Darnest Things
31. The Hee ............................. Haw Show
32. The Beverly .........................Hillbillies
33. Gilligan's....................................Island
34. Beat The ................................. Clock
35. Sesame........................................Street
36. WLS..............................Barn Dance

# PERSONS IN SONG
CREATED BY GLENN SEYMOUR

1.  When You And I Were Young .................................................................

2.  If You Knew................................................................. Like I Knew

3.  Take Me Home Again ..........................................................................

4.  .................................................................Give Me Your Answer True

5.  Wait Til The Sun Shines..................................................................

6.  Sweet ..................................................................................................

7.  My Own..............................................................................................

8.  .................................................................................Blue Gown

9.  Good Night ..........................................................................................

10.  .................................................................Sweet as Apple Cider

11.  .................................................................Won't You Blow Your Horn

12.  ................................................................................. Don't cry

13.  Sweet ..................................................................... ,my Adeline

14.  Does Your Mother Know You're Out..........................................................

15.  Won't You Come Home ......................................................................

16.  Oh.................................................................Don't You Cry For Me

17.  Hang Down Your Head ........................................................................

18.  My Wild Irish...................................................................................

# PERSONS IN SONG
## CREATED BY GLENN SEYMOUR

1. When You and I Were Young .......................................................................... Maggie

2. If You knew .......................................................... Susie......Like I knew.......Susie

3. Take Me Home Again ......................................................................... Kathleen

4. Daisy, Daisy ......................................................... Give Me Your Answer True

5. Wait Til The Sun Shines............................................................................Nellie

6. Sweet ..................................................................................................Sue

7. My Own.............................................................................................Iona

8. Alice ........................................................................................Blue Gown

9. Good Night ......................................................................................Irene

10. Ida.......................................................................... Sweet As Apple Cider

11. Dinah ....................................................... Won't You Blow Your Horn

12. Toot Toot Tootsie......................................................................... Don't Cry

13. Sweet ....................................................... Adeline, my Adeline

14. Does Your Mother Know You're Out................................................Cecilia

15. Won't You Come Home...........................................................Bill Bailey

16. Oh Susanna ....................................................... Don't You Cry For Me

17. Hang Down Your Head ........................................................... Tom Dooley

18. My Wild Irish.................................................................................Rose

# PRODUCT NAMES

# WHAT IS IT? 1
## CREATED BY GLENN SEYMOUR

1.   Bounce .................................................................................................

2.   Loafer ..................................................................................................

3.   Cottonelle ...........................................................................................

4.   Windex ...............................................................................................

5.   Rolltop ...............................................................................................

6.   Ruben .................................................................................................

7.   Shafer .................................................................................................

8.   One A Day ..........................................................................................

9.   Samsonite ..........................................................................................

10.  Pullover .............................................................................................

11.  Grit ....................................................................................................

12.  Webster ..............................................................................................

13.  Dole ...................................................................................................

14.  Stetson ...............................................................................................

15.  Fez .....................................................................................................

16.  Imperial .............................................................................................

17.  Beauty Rest ........................................................................................

18.  Lazy Boy ............................................................................................

19.  Turkish ...............................................................................................

20.  Smith Bros ..........................................................................................

21.  Kelly ..................................................................................................

22.  Naval ..................................................................................................

23.  Nutmeg ..............................................................................................

24.  Vidalia................................................................................................

# WHAT IS IT? 1
CREATED BY GLENN SEYMOUR

1.   Bounce .............................................................................. fabric softener

2.   Loafer ........................................................................................ shoe

3.   Cottonelle ....................................................................... toilet tissue

4.   Windex ............................................................................ glass cleaner

5.   Roll top .................................................................................... desk

6.   Ruben ................................................................................. sandwich

7.   Shafer ............................................................................ fountain pen

8.   One A Day ............................................................................. vitamin

9.   Samsonite ............................................................................ luggage

10.  Pullover ............................................................................... sweater

11.  Grit ................................................................................. newspaper

12.  Webster ............................................................................ dictionary

13   Dole .................................................................................. pineapple

14.  Stetson ...................................................................................... hat

15.  Fez ........................................................................................... cap

16.  Imperial .................................................................................... oleo

17.  Beauty Rest ......................................................................... mattress

18.  Lazy Boy ............................................................................ furniture

19.  Turkish .................................................................................. towel

20.  Smith Bros ...................................................................... cough drops

21.  Kelly ............................................................................... potato chips

22.  Naval .................................................................................... orange

23.  Nutmeg .................................................................................. spice

24.  Vidalie .................................................................................... onion

# WHAT IS IT? 2
### CREATED BY GLENN SEYMOUR

1. Dinty Moore _____

2. Vixen _____

3. Chicken Noodle _____

4. Rambler _____

5. Roaring animal _____

6. Door lock _____

7. Adder _____

8. Drone _____

9. Slicker _____

10. Big Boy _____

11. Egg drink _____

12. Poland China _____

13. Nova _____

14. Drake _____

15. Maiden Blush _____

16. Cub _____

17. Cornish _____

18. Night flyers _____

19. Nylons _____

20. Cashew _____

21. Long legged bird _____

22. Butterball _____

23. Rodent _____

24. Tube _____

25. Leaf or head _____

26. RedWing _____

27. Truck for moving _____

28. Small singing bird _____

29. Scavenger bird _____

30. Striped animal _____

31. Black widow _____

32. Blue racer _____

33. Razor backs _____

34. Hooter _____

35. Vidalia _____

36. Pippin _____

# WHAT IS IT? 2
## CREATED BY GLENN SEYMOUR

1. Dinty Moore ......................beef stew
2. Vixen ...............................fox
3. Chicken Noodle ....................soup
4. Rambler..............................car
5. Roaring animal...........................lion
6. Door lock ...............................key
7. Adder................................ snake
8. Drone............................. male bee
9. Slicker ..........................rain coat
10. Big Boy ...........................tomato
11. Egg drink ......................... egg nogg
12. Poland China................................ hog
13. Nova ................................car
14. Drake............................. duck
15. Maiden Blush ......................apple
16. Cub ..........................baby bear
17. Cornish ......................... hen
18. Nght flyers................................bats

19. Nylons ...................................stockings
20. Cashew.............................. nut
21. Long legged bird ...................... stork
22. Butterball ...............................turkey
23. Rodent............................. mouse - rat
24. Tube ................................ socks
25. Leaf or head ........................... lettuce
26. RedWing................................... shoes
27. Truck for moving.......................van
28. Small singing bird........canary - wren
29. Scavenger bird.......................buzzard
30. Striped animal...........................zebra
31. Black widow.............................. spider
32. Blue racer ................................ snake
33. Razor backs.............................hogs
34. Hooter ..............................owl
35. Vidalia ...........................onion
36. Pippin ...............................apple

154

# BRAND NAME PRODUCTS
CREATED BY GLENN SEYMOUR

1.  Palmolive _____
2.  Edsel _____
3.  Zenith _____
4.  Nikon _____
5.  Corelle _____
6.  Hoover _____
7.  Hanes _____
8.  Pringles _____
9.  Wrangler _____
10. London Fog _____
11. Longhorn _____
12. Samsonite _____
13. Imperial _____
14. Timex _____
15. Beauty Rest _____
16. Lawn Boy _____
17. Maytag _____
18. Roper _____
19. John Deere _____
20. Goodyear _____
21. Bissell _____
22. Remington _____
23. Stetson _____
24. Ball or Kerr _____
25. Rival _____
26. Skippy _____
27. Quaker State _____
28. Sanka _____
29. Welch _____
30. Singer _____
31. Schwinn _____
32. Alpo _____
33. Polaroid _____
34. Wolverine _____
35. Dutch Boy _____
36. Skil _____
37. Naturalizer _____
38. Cold Spot _____
39. Royal _____
40. Bunn _____
41. Red Wing _____
42. Bell _____
43. Black & Decker _____
44. Kelly _____
45. Campbell _____
46. Bic _____
47. McCormick _____
48. Quasar _____
49. Aladdin _____
50. 1-2 Opaline _____

# BRAND NAME PRODUCTS
## CREATED BY GLENN SEYMOUR

| | | |
|---|---|---|
| 1. | Palmolive | soap |
| 2. | Edsel | car |
| 3. | Zenith | TV |
| 4. | Nikon | camera |
| 5. | Corelle | dishes |
| 6. | Hoover | vacuum cleaner |
| 7. | Hanes | underwear |
| 8. | Pringles | potato chips |
| 9. | Wrangler | jeans |
| 10. | London Fog | coat |
| 11. | Longhorn | cheese |
| 12. | Samsonite | luggage |
| 13. | Imperial | oleo |
| 14. | Timex | watch |
| 15. | Beauty Rest | mattress |
| 16. | Lawn Boy | lawnmower |
| 17. | Maytag | washer - dryer |
| 18. | Roper | stove |
| 19. | John Deere | tractor |
| 20. | Goodyear | tires |
| 21. | Bissell | sweeper |
| 22. | Remington | razor |
| 23. | Stetson | hat |
| 24. | Ball or Kerr | canning supplies |
| 25. | Rival | dog food |
| 26. | Skippy | peanut butter |
| 27. | Quaker State | motor oil |
| 28. | Sanka | coffee |
| 29. | Welch | juice - jam - jelly |
| 30. | Singer | sewing machine |
| 31. | Schwinn | bicycle |
| 32. | Alpo | dog food |
| 33. | Polaroid | camera |
| 34. | Wolverine | shoes |
| 35. | Dutch Boy | cleanser |
| 36. | Skil | saw |
| 37. | Naturalizer | shoe |
| 38. | Cold Spot | refrigerator |
| 39. | Royal | typewriter |
| 40. | Bunn | coffee pot |
| 41. | Red Wing | shoes |
| 42. | Bell | telephone |
| 43. | Black & Decker | tools |
| 44. | Kelly | potato chips |
| 45. | Campbell | soup |
| 46. | Bic | pens |
| 47. | McCormick | spices |
| 48. | Quasar | TV |
| 49. | Aladdin | lamp |
| 50. | 1-2 Opaline | oil |

# FIRST & LAST WORDS 1
## CREATED BY GLENN SEYMOUR

1. Elmer's .......................................................................................................

2. Corelle .......................................................................................................

3. SOS .......................................................................................................

4. Niagara .......................................................................................................

5. Royal Blue .......................................................................................................

6. Corning Ware .......................................................................................................

7. Sunbeam .......................................................................................................

8. Bo Peep .......................................................................................................

9. Smith Bros .......................................................................................................

10. Old English .......................................................................................................

11. Efferdent .......................................................................................................

12. Rit .......................................................................................................

13. Grandfather .......................................................................................................

14. Coldspot .......................................................................................................

15. Chiquita .......................................................................................................

16. Pam .......................................................................................................

17. Glidden .......................................................................................................

18. Karo .......................................................................................................

# FIRST & LAST WORDS 1
CREATED BY GLENN SEYMOUR

1. Elmer's ........................................................................................... glue

2. Corelle ....................................................................................dinnerware

3. SOS ....................................................................................... soap pad

4. Niagara ...................................................................................... starch

5. Royal Blue ....................................................................................bluing

6. Corning Ware ..........................................................................oven ware

7. Sunbeam ......................................................................................bread

8. Bo Peep ...................................................................................ammonia

9. Smith Bros ...........................................................................cough drops

10. Old English............................................................................ furniture polish

11. Efferdent .........................................................................denture cleaner

12. Rit ...............................................................................................dye

13. Grandfather............................................................................... clock

14. Coldspot ...............................................................................refrigerator

15. Chiquita ....................................................................................banana

16. Pam........................................................................................ cooking spray

17. Glidden .......................................................................................paint

18. Karo..........................................................................................syrup

# FIRST & LAST WORDS 2
### CREATED BY GLENN SEYMOUR

1.  SOS _____

2.  COPPER Glo_____

3.  Royal Blue _____

4.  Corning_____

5.  Bopeep _____

6.  Dow_____

7.  Raid_____

8.  Rit _____

9.  Old English _____

10. Miracle Gro_____

11. Grandfather_____

12. Coldspot _____

13. Mixmaster_____

14. Masking _____

15. Heinz_____

16. Calumet_____

17. Jimmy Dean _____

18. Karo _____

19. Star Kist_____

20. Idaho_____

21. Vadalia _____

22. French's _____

23. Glazed _____

24. Chocolate Chip _____

25. Graham _____

26. Sunbeam _____

27. Lipton _____

28. Smith Brothers _____

29. Bufferin_____

# FIRST AND LAST WORDS 2
CREATED BY GLENN SEYMOUR

1.  SOS ................................................................ scouring pads
2.  COPPER Glo ..................................................... polish
3.  Royal Blue ...................................................... bluing
4.  Corning ........................................................... oven ware
5.  Bopeep ........................................................... ammonia
6.  Dow ............................................................... oven cleaner
7.  Raid .............................................................. bug killer
8.  Rit ................................................................ dye
9.  Old English ..................................................... furniture polish
10. Miracle Gro ..................................................... fertilizer
11. Grandfather ..................................................... clock
12. Coldspot ......................................................... refrigerator
13. Mixmaster ....................................................... mixer
14. Masking .......................................................... tape
15. Heinz ............................................................. catsup
16. Calumet .......................................................... baking soda
17. Jimmy Dean ...................................................... sausage
18. Karo .............................................................. syrup
19. Star Kist ........................................................ tuna
20. Idaho ............................................................. potato
21. Vadalia .......................................................... onion
22. French's ......................................................... mustard
23. Glazed ........................................................... doughnuts
24. Chocolate Chip ................................................. cookies
25. Graham ........................................................... crackers
26. Sunbeam ......................................................... bread-buns
27. Lipton ............................................................ tea
28. Smith Brothers .................................................. caugh drops
29. Bufferin .......................................................... aspirin

# SCHOOL

# GRADE SCHOOL - SOME GOLDEN DAYS
## CREATED BY GLENN SEYMOUR

1. School in early days? .............................................................................
2. Source of water at school? ........................................................................
3. What did they use for a toilet? ..................................................................
4. What was inside the front door? ................................................................
5. How many grades taught? ........................................................................
6. How are grades kept? ...............................................................................
7. How are parents informed of grades? ........................................................
8. Where were classes recited? ......................................................................
9. How was school heated? ...........................................................................
10. What were the other buildings? ...............................................................
11. What was the groove in the upper part of the desk used for? .....................
........................................................................................................................
12. What was the glass cup in upper right corner of desk? ..............................
13. Where were the books kept? .....................................................................
14. What was the name of the writing method? ...............................................
15. What competitive games were played between schools? ............................
16. One outstanding program per year? .........................................................
17. Who helped the Teacher with water and fuel? ..........................................
18. Where you passed from one grade to another? .........................................
19. How did you get to school? ......................................................................
20. Later how did you get to school? ..............................................................
21. What games did the children play? ...........................................................
22. How are classes divided now? ..................................................................
23. Do they have competitive sports? .............................................................
24. Name one popular sport? .........................................................................
25. Do students have cold lunches? ................................................................
26. Where do they get hot meals? ..................................................................
27. Who is the Teachers Supervisor? ..............................................................
28. Schools are controlled by? ........................................................................
29. What is the class for 5 year olds? ..............................................................
30. What age do they enter grade school? .......................................................
31. Upon graduation what do they receive? ....................................................
32. What does this entitle you to? ...................................................................

# GRADE SCHOOL - SOME GOLDEN DAYS
### CREATED BY GLENN SEYMOUR

1.   School in early days? .......................................... one room country school
2.   Source of water at school? ........................well - water bucket and dipper
3.   What did they use for a toilet? .............. privies out back for boys & girls
4.   What was inside the front door? ..................................................cloak room
5.   How many grades taught? ............................................................................ 8
6.   How are grades kept? ..................................................................report card
7.   How are parents informed of grades?...........cards are sent home, signed and returned
8.   Where were classes recited? .....................................on a bench up front
9.   How was school heated?...........................coal or cob stove in the corner
10.  What were the other buildings? ....... carriage house for horse & buggies
11.  What was the groove in the upper part of the desk used for? ..........place for pens and pencils
12.  What was the glass cup in upper right corner of desk?.................ink well
13.  Where were the books kept? .......................................................in the desk
14.  What was the name of the writing method?................................. palmer
15.  What competitive games were played between schools? ..................none
16.  One outstanding program per year ......................................... Christmas
17.  Who helped the Teacher with water and fuel? ........................ upper class
18.  Where you passed from one grade to another?......................... promoted
19.  How did you get to school?...................................... walked - rode a horse
20.  Later how did you get to school?............................... walked - rode a bus
21.  What games did the children play?......... tag - ball - fly kites - Blackman
22.  How are classes divided now?...................................one class per room
23.  Do they have competitive sports? ............................................................ yes
24.  Name one popular sport?............................ football - basketball - soccer
25.  Do students have cold lunches?.................................................................no
26.  Where do they get hot meals? ......................................................cafeteria
27.  Who are the Teachers Supervisor?...................................Superintendent
28.  Schools are controlled by?..............................................elected board
29.  What is the class for 5 year olds?....................................kindergarten
30.  What age do they enter grade school?.................................................six
31.  Upon graduation what do they receive?.......................................diploma
32.  What does this entitle you to? .....................................enter high school

# HIGH SCHOOL
## CREATED BY GLENN SEYMOUR

1. How many years of school?..................................................................................

2. Name the years. ......................................................................................................

3. How many subjects must you take every year? ...............................................

4. What does each subject equal? ..........................................................................

5. How many credits needed to graduate? ...........................................................

6. Are certain subjects required to enter College?..............................................

7. Where do you spend time when not in class? ..................................................

8. What do you receive upon graduation? ............................................................

9. Name some competitive sports. ........................................................................

10. One popular girls sports are..............................................................................

11. Students eat lunch in the ...................................................................................

12. Name two outdoor sports. ..................................................................................

13. Name two indoor sports.......................................................................................

14. What may a student that excels in grades receive? ........................................

# HIGH SCHOOL
## CREATED BY GLENN SEYMOUR

1. How many years of school?................................................................................4

2. Name the years ..................................................Freshman, Sophomore, Junior, Senior

3. How many subjects must you take every year? ................................................at least 4

4. What does each subject equal? .......................................................... one credit

5. How many credits needed to graduate? ...................................................... 16

6. Are certain subjects required to enter College?......................................... yes

7. Where do you spend time when not in class? ....................................study hall

8. What do you receive upon graduation? .......................................... diploma

9. Name some competitive sports?.........................................football, basketball, soccer

10. One popular girls sports are?..............................................soccer, basketball, volleyball

11. Students eat lunch in the ........................................................................cafeteria

12. Name two outdoor sports?...................................................... football, soccer

13. Name two indoor sports?........................................................ basketball, volleyball

14. What may a student that excels in grades receive? .................. Scholarship to College

# COLLEGE
## CREATED BY GLENN SEYMOUR

1.  What is a college fee called? _____

2.  Students living quarters are called? _____

3.  Ladies organization? _____

4.  Mens organization? _____

5.  What are the grounds called? _____

6.  Shortest number of years to get a degree? _____

7.  Name two competitive sports _____

8.  Where do winning teams go? _____

9.  Name three bowls. _____

10. What is the experimental room called? _____

11. What is the reference room called? _____

12. Name the mascot of University of Illinois. _____

13. Where are football games played? _____

14. Where are basketball games played? _____

15. What is the list for honor students? _____

16. What do some Universities call the first week? _____

17. What are loans for students called? _____

18. Where is one branch of University of Illinois located? _____

19. What are gifts for students to help pay tuition? _____

# COLLEGE
## CREATED BY GLENN SEYMOUR

1.  What is a college fee called? .............................................................tuition

2.  Students living quarters are called? ...............................................dormitories

3.  Ladies organization? ......................................................................sorority

4.  Mens organization? .......................................................................fraternity

5.  What are the grounds called? .........................................................campus

6.  Shortest number of years to get a degree? ................................................. 4

7.  Name two competitive sports ...............................................football - basketball

8.  Where do winning teams go? ........................................................bowl games

9.  Name three bowls................................................................Rose - Sugar - Orange

10. What is the experimental room called?.......................................... laboratory

11. What is the reference room called?...............................................library

12. Name the mascot of University of Illinois..............................Chief Illiniwik

13. Where are football games played?.................................................. stadium

14. Where are basketball games played?...........................................gymnasium

15. What is the list for honor students? ............................................ Deans list

16. What do some Universities call the first week? ................................ Freshmen week

17. What are loans for students called?.........................................Student loans

18. Where is one branch of University of Illinois located? ............................. Springfield

19. What are gifts for students to help pay tuition? .........................................scholarships

# WORDS

# MISSING WORDS
CREATED BY GLENN SEYMOUR

1. _____ Carte

2. _____ Arbor, Michigan

3. Dinah _____

4. Tea for _____

5. _____ got a Secret

6. Flight of The _____

7. Last of The _____

8. Yes, We Have No _____

9. White Cliffs of _____

10. _____ sound

11. Out And _____

12. _____ and downs

13. The _____ Ranger

14. Mutiny on The _____

15. Alma_____

16. Much Ado About _____

17. Trick or_____

18. How Deep is The _____

19. Robert E _____

20. Meet Me In _____

21. To Kill A _____

22. To See Is To _____

23. Still Water Runs _____

24. Suit To A_____

25. Mad As A Wet _____

26. All Around The _____

27. All Is Well That Ends _____

28. Ode To _____

29. I'm A Little _____

30. Walking The Floor _____

# MISSING WORDS
CREATED BY GLENN SEYMOUR

1. Ala................................ carte

2. Ann...................... Arbor, Michigan

3. Dinah........................... Shore

4. Tea For.......................... Two

5. I've.....................Got A Secret

6. Flight of The .................. Bumblebee

7. Last of The ..................Mohicans

8. Yes, We Have No ................ Bananas

9. White Cliffs Of...................... Dover

10. Puget..........................Sound

11. Out and ........................ About

12. Ups........................and downs

13. The ................Lone .......Ranger

14. Mutiny on The..................... Bounty

15. Alma ...........................Mater

16. Much Ado About................ Nothing

17. Trick or.......................... Treat

18. How Deep Is the ..................... Ocean

19. Robert E. ...........................Lee

20. Meet Me In .......................... St. Louis

21. To Kill A.......................Mocking Bird

22. To see is to ............................believe

23. Still water runs ...........................deep

24. Suit to a ...............................tee

25. Mad as a wet................................. hen

26. All Around the ......... Mulberry Bush

27. All is well that ends....................... well

28. Ode To.................................. Billie Jo

29. I'm A Little..............................Teapot

30. Walking the Floor............. Over You

172

# WORDS USED TWO WAYS - SOME ARE SLANG 1

CREATED BY GLENN SEYMOUR

1. Aim _____     aim _____

2. Air _____     air _____

3. Alarm _____     alarm _____

4. Ace _____     ace _____

5. Arm _____     arm _____

6. Ape _____     ape _____

7. Axe _____     axe _____

8. Attack _____     attack _____

9. Admit _____     admit _____

10. Angle _____     angle _____

11. Abide _____     abide _____

12. Article _____     article _____

13. Appendix _____     appendix _____

14. Ash _____     ash _____

15. Bangs _____     bangs _____

16. Base _____     base _____

17. Beat _____     beat _____

# WORDS USED TWO WAYS - SOME ARE SLANG 1
## CREATED BY GLENN SEYMOUR

1. Aim.............................point a gun     aim...................................in life

2. Air...............................atmosphere     air....................................by radio

3. Alarm.......................part of a clock     alarm..............................scare - frighten

4. Ace....................................high card     ace....................................best aviator

5. Arm........................part of the body     arm..........................outfit an army

6. Ape........................................animal     ape.............................mock - copy

7. Axe...........................................tool     axe................................fire a person

8. Attack..........................heart attack     attack.................. using force on a person

9. Admit.......................allow to enter     admit..................................confess

10. Angle......................fish with a hook     angle.............................a different view

11. Abide..........................................live     abide.........................obey the rules

12. Article.....................................object     article............................piece in the paper

13. Appendix.............part of the body     appendix..............................index - listing

14. Ash............................................tree     ash...................................fire residue

15. Bang.................................loud noise     bangs.............................hair style

16. Base....................................foundation     base...........................first stop in baseball

17. Beat..........................................whip     beat...................................overcome

# WORDS USED TWO WAYS - SOME ARE SLANG 2
## CREATED BY GLENN SEYMOUR

18. Bind _____  bind _____

19. Bag _____  bag _____

20. Box _____  box _____

21. Bum _____  bum _____

22. Bat _____  bat _____

23. Beam _____  beam _____

24. Boil _____  boil _____

25. Bark _____  bark _____

26. Bank _____  bank _____

27. Boat _____  boat _____

28. Bit _____  bit _____

29. Brand _____  brand _____

30. Bed _____  bed _____

31. Bunk _____  bunk _____

32. Bowl _____  bowl _____

33. Bridge _____  bridge _____

34. Crop _____  crop _____

35. Coast _____  coast _____

# WORDS USED TWO WAYS - SOME ARE SLANG 2
## CREATED BY GLENN SEYMOUR

| | | | |
|---|---|---|---|
| 18. | Bind................................................tie | bind...........................get in a bad situation |
| 19. | Bag..............................................container | bag..............................taking of wild game |
| 20. | Box ............................................container | box.........................................................fight |
| 21. | Bum.......................................... hobo | bum ............................................... bad rap |
| 22. | Bat.......................................mammal | bat......................................used to hit a ball |
| 23. | Beam .............................. shine light | beam.......................................ceiling timber |
| 24. | Boil ....................................infection | boil.........................................................to heat |
| 25. | Bark ........................... part of a tree | bark............................... sound a dog makes |
| 26. | Bank ...................... side of a stream | bank....................money exchanging place |
| 27. | Boat ............................sailing vessel | boat............................. in a bad situation |
| 28. | Bit ............................. small amount | bit............................................ boring tool |
| 29. | Brand.......................................mark | brand...........................name of a product |
| 30. | Bed.............................place to sleep | bed........................................plot of flowers |
| 31. | Bunk...............................talk wildly | bunk ............. a bed on top of another bed |
| 32. | Bowl .............................................dish | bowl.......where football games are played |
| 33. | Bridge......................span a river | bridge ............................................card game |
| 34. | Crop ........................................ to cut | crop........................... what land produces |
| 35. | Coast ............................ shoreline | coast................................................free wheel |

# WORDS USED TWO WAYS - SOME ARE SLANG 3

CREATED BY GLENN SEYMOUR

1.  Can _____    can _____

2.  Clod _____    clod _____

3.  Coat _____    coat _____

4.  Cram _____    cram _____

5.  Club _____    club _____

6.  Cord _____    cord _____

7.  Card _____    card _____

8.  Coin _____    coin _____

9.  Creep _____    creep _____

10.  Crank _____    crank _____

11.  Cold _____    cold _____

12.  Clam _____    clam _____

13.  Couple _____    couple _____

14.  Crowd _____    crowd _____

15.  Crib _____    crib _____

16.  Cool _____    cool _____

17.  Cape _____    cape _____

18.  Crook _____    crook _____

# WORDS USED TWO WAYS - SOME ARE SLANG 3
## CREATED BY GLENN SEYMOUR

1. Can ............................. able     can ........................... preserve

2. Clod.....................lump of soil     clod............................. worthless person

3. Coat.........................cover     Coat............................. wearing apparel

4. Cram .....................pack tightly     cram............................. study for exam

5. Club........................a group     club.............................heavy stick

6. Cord ........................ string     cord............................. measurer of wood

7. Card.........................message     card.............................lively person

8. Coin........................ money     coin............................. to say a phrase

9. Creep................. move very slowly     creep............................. odd person

10. Crank ................. part of an old car     crank............................disagreeable person

11. Cold............................ lack of heat     cold............................. chest infection

12. Clam.........................seafood     clam............................. refuses to speak

13. Couple.........................two people     couple............................join together

14. Crowd ........................ shove - push     crowd............................group

15. Crib ................. place to store corn     crib............................. baby bed

16. Cool.........................a calm person     cool............................. not hot or cold

17. Cape ................. place in the ocean     cape............................. garment

18. Crook ................. place in the road     crook ............................. dishonest person

# WORDS USED TWO WAYS - SOME ARE SLANG 4
CREATED BY GLENN SEYMOUR

1. Cell _____     cell _____

2. Comb _____     comb _____

3. Clutch _____     clutch _____

4. Dab _____     dab _____

5. Dodge _____     dodge _____

6. Date _____     date _____

7. Dough _____     dough _____

8. Dart _____     dart _____

9. Deed _____     deed _____

10. Dead _____     dead _____

11. Drop _____     drop _____

12. Drum _____     drum _____

13. Dig _____     dig _____

14. Doze _____     doze _____

15. Dump _____     dump _____

16. Dust _____     dust _____

17. Ditch _____     ditch _____

18. Draft _____     draft _____

# WORDS USED TWO WAYS - SOME ARE SLANG 4
## CREATED BY GLENN SEYMOUR

1. Cell ............................. blood          cell ............................. room in a prison
2. Comb ................. used in hair care          comb ......................... top of a rooster's head
3. Clutch ............................. grasp          clutch ............................. part of a car
4. Dab ........................ small amount          dab ......................... splatters as on a wall
5. Dodge ............................. car          dodge ............................. evade
6. Date ........................ an appointment          date ........................ day on the calendar
7. Dough ............................. money          dough ............................. pastries
8. Dart ........................ move quickly          dart ............. pointed object used in games
9. Deed ............................. title          deed ............................. a good act
10. Dead ............................. lifeless          dead ............................. end of a street
11. Drop ............................. wee bit          drop ............................. let fall
12. Drum ............. musical instrument          drum ......................... part of a car
13. Dig ............................. move soil          dig ............................. understanding
14. Doze ............................. nap          doze ............................. dig out a tree
15. Dump ............................. unload          dump ........................ old dilapidated house
16. Dust ................. particles in the air          dust ............................. clean furniture
17. Ditch ................. where water flows          ditch ............................. get rid of
18. Draft ............................. air flow          draft ......................... call to armed forces

# WORDS USED TWO WAYS - SOME ARE SLANG 5

CREATED BY GLENN SEYMOUR

1. Dice _____    dice _____

2. Deck _____    deck _____

3. Drill _____    drill _____

4. Dane _____    dane _____

5. Draw _____    draw _____

6. Dwell _____    dwell _____

7. Drift _____    drift _____

8. Dutch _____    dutch _____

9. Even _____    even _____

10. Eat _____    eat _____

11. Edge _____    edge _____

12. Engage _____    engage _____

13. Extra _____    extra _____

14. Elder _____    elder _____

15. Ear _____    ear _____

16. Eye _____    eye _____

17. Egg _____    egg _____

# WORDS USED TWO WAYS - SOME ARE SLANG 5
## CREATED BY GLENN SEYMOUR

1. Dice ...................... gambling cubes    dice ................................ cut in small pieces

2. Deck ...................floor of a boat    deck ..........................................playing cards

3. Drill.............................. tool    drill........................................military act

4. Dane......................breed of a dog    dane.......................person from Denmark

5. Draw........................... sketch    draw....................... draw a crowd

6. Dwell............................reside    dwell .......... talk constantly on one subject

7. Drift............................ pile of snow    drift................................ to wander

8. Dutch ..........each pay his own way    dutch ........................ person from Holland

9. Even....................tied in score    even ..........................................level

10. Eat.......................consume    eat ............................... away as erode

11. Edge...............................rim    edge .................................advantaage

12. Engage...............................take part    engage ................................ purpose to wed

13. Extra........................... spare    extra........................ additional newspaper

14. Elder......................head of Church    elder........................................ tree

15. Ear ........................ part of the body    ear ............................part of a stalk of corn

16. Eye ........................ part of the body    eye................................center of hurricane

17. Egg............................ food    egg ............................urge someone to act

# WORDS USED TWO WAYS - SOME ARE SLANG 6
## CREATED BY GLENN SEYMOUR

1.   Embrace _____          embrace _____

2.   Ebony _____            ebony _____

3.   Elevate _____          elevate _____

4.   Fan_____               fan_____

5.   Fit _____              fit_____

6.   Faint _____            faint_____

7.   Foot_____              foot _____

8.   Fade_____              fade _____

9.   Fog_____               fog_____

10.  Fix _____              fix _____

11.  Flat _____             flat_____

12.  Face _____             face _____

13.  Fire _____             fire_____

14.  Figure _____           figure_____

15.  Ford_____              ford _____

16.  Fork_____              fork _____

17.  Gag _____              gag _____

# WORDS USED TWO WAYS - SOME ARE SLANG 6
### CREATED BY GLENN SEYMOUR

1. Embrace...........................hug — embrace...........................to accept
2. Ebony...........................black — ebony...........................wood
3. Elevate...........................lift — elevate...........................promote
4. Fan...........................stir air — fan...........................follower of sports
5. Fit...........................correct — fit...........................a tantrum
6. Faint...........................pass out — faint...........................dim
7. Foot...........................12 inches — foot...........................part of the body
8. Fade...........................disappear — fade...........................lose color
9. Fog...........................mist — fog...........................state of confusion
10. Fix...........................repair — fix...........................in trouble
11. Flat...........................musical term — flat...........................living quarters
12. Face...........................front of a clock — face...........................part of the body
13. Fire...........................something burning — fire...........................dismiss from a job
14. Figure...........................shape — figure...........................to calculate
15. Ford...........................car — ford...........................cross a creek
16. Fork...........................eating utensil — fork...........................when the road divides
17. Gag...........................joke — gag...........................Silence - muffle

# WORDS USED TWO WAYS - SOME ARE SLANG 7

CREATED BY GLENN SEYMOUR

1. Grain_____ grain _____

2. Goat _____ goat _____

3. Grip_____ grip _____

4. Game_____ game _____

5. Goal_____ goal _____

6. Grub _____ grub _____

7. Gums_____ gums _____

8. Gift _____ gift _____

9. Grind_____ grind _____

10. Gear _____ gear _____

11. Gander _____ gander _____

12. Haze _____ haze _____

13. Harp _____ harp _____

14. Hit_____ hit _____

15. Ham _____ ham _____

16. Hug_____ hug_____

17. Hamper_____ hamper _____

# WORDS USED TWO WAYS - SOME ARE SLANG 7
### CREATED BY GLENN SEYMOUR

1.  Grain ............................... farm crop
    grain ........................................ particle of salt

2.  Goat............................... animal
    goat ........................................ get one angry

3.  Grip .............................. illness
    grip .........................................hold hand tight

4.  Game............................contest
    game ........................................ wild animal

5.  Goal..............................aim in life
    goal ....................................score in football

6.  Grub .............................. food
    grub .............................. dugout as a stump

7.  Gums................. part of the mouth
    gums...................................... chewing gum

8.  Gift................................a present
    gift............................................ special ability

9.  Grind............................ sharpen
    grind....................same thing day after day

10. Gear .............................clothing
    gear ............................................ part of a car

11. Grander.........................male goose
    gander ............................... take a look

12. Haze ...............................fog
    haze............................... to punish

13. Harp ............... musical instrument
    harp ...........................talk on same subject

14. Hit.................................strike
    hit....................................popular as a song

15. Ham............................ hog meat
    ham....................................... actor

16. Hug...............................embrace
    hug................................ ride the center line

17. Hamper.........................bother
    hamper...........................place for clothes

# WORDS USED TWO WAYS - SOME ARE SLANG 8
## CREATED BY GLENN SEYMOUR

1. Host_____ host_____

2. Hack _____ hack _____

3. Hose _____ hose_____

4. Hide_____ hide_____

5. Horn _____ horn _____

6. Hound_____ hound _____

7. Iron _____ iron _____

8. Ice _____ ice _____

9. Idle _____ idle _____

10. Ivy _____ ivy_____

11. Inclined _____ inclined_____

12. Implement_____ implement_____

13. Ivory _____ ivory _____

14. Index _____ index_____

15. Inquire_____ inquire _____

16. Item _____ item_____

17. Inch _____ inch_____

18. Iris _____ iris_____

# WORDS USED TWO WAYS - SOME ARE SLANG 8
## CREATED BY GLENN SEYMOUR

1. Host......................entertainer
   host......................great number of things

2. Hack......................cut - chop
   hack......................taxi cab

3. Hose......................nylon stockings
   hose......................tube for sending water

4. Hide......................conceal
   hide......................animal coat

5. Horn......................musical instrument
   horn......................found on cows head

6. Hound......................dog
   hound......................pester

7. Iron......................metal
   iron......................press clothes

8. Ice......................frozen water
   ice......................frost a cake

9. Idle......................unemployed
   idle......................run a motor slowly

10. Ivy......................vine
    ivy......................Ivy league School

11. Inclined......................sloped
    inclined......................to follow the crowd

12. Implement......................tool
    implement......................enforce

13. Ivory......................color
    ivory......................elephant tusks

14. Index......................to file
    index......................directory

15. Inquire......................magazine
    inquire......................ask

16. Item......................news
    item......................one thing on a list

17. Inch......................a measure
    inch......................move slowly

18. Iris......................flower
    iris......................part of the eye

# WORDS USED TWO WAYS - SOME ARE SLANG 9
### CREATED BY GLENN SEYMOUR

1. Jingle _____    jingle _____

2. Joker _____    joker _____

3. Jaw _____    jaw _____

4. Jug _____    jug _____

5. Joint _____    joint _____

6. Jam _____    jam _____

7. Juice _____    juice _____

8. Jar _____    jar _____

9. Jack _____    jack _____

10. Jog _____    jog _____

11. Jet _____    jet _____

12. King _____    king _____

13. Key _____    key _____

14. Kid _____    kid _____

15. Knot _____    knot _____

16. Kill _____    kill _____

17. Kinky _____    kinky _____

# WORDS USED TWO WAYS - SOME ARE SLANG 9

CREATED BY GLENN SEYMOUR

1. Jingle ............................... ring          jingle ............................... short poem
2. Joker .......................... trick player          joker ........................ in a deck of cards
3. Jaw ........................ part of the head          jaw .............................. a friendly chat
4. Jug .................................. container          jug .......................................... in jail
5. Joint ....... two things that are joined          joint ..................... small eating place
6. Jam .................................... food          jam ............................... traffic tie up
7. Juice ................................ drink          juice ...................... life in a battery
8. Jar ............................... sudden jolt          jar ................................... container
9. Jack ................................ car lift          jack ......................... a playing card
10. Jog .................... curve in a road          jog .......................... a walking pace
11. Jet ............................... airplane          jet ...................................... black
12. King ................. ruler of a country          king ........................ a playing card
13. Key ........................... on a piano          key ............... used to unlock a door
14. Kid ............................ baby goat          kid .................................... torment
15. Knot .................................. tie          knot ...................... burl in a board
16. Kill .................................. slay          kill .......................... pass time away
17. Kinky ............................ weird          kinky ...................... curly as in hair

# WORDS USED TWO WAYS - SOME ARE SLANG 10
## CREATED BY GLENN SEYMOUR

1.  Kitty_____    kitty_____

2.  Knit _____    knit _____

3.  Knob _____    knob _____

4.  Lap_____    lap_____

5.  Loaf _____    loaf _____

6.  Land _____    land_____

7.  Log _____    log_____

8.  Link_____    link _____

9.  Left _____    left_____

10. Limb _____    limb_____

11. Lace_____    lace _____

12. Lead_____    lead _____

13. Level _____    level_____

14. Lord_____    lord _____

15. Leaf _____    leaf _____

16. Last _____    last _____

17. Lodge_____    lodge _____

# WORDS USED TWO WAYS - SOME ARE SLANG 10
## CREATED BY GLENN SEYMOUR

1.  Kitty............................... cat | kitty ...................................... jackpot
2.  Knit.................................heal | knit ...............................form of crochet
3.  Knob........................... door handle | knob ................................... mound of dirt
4.  Lap..................................fold over | lap ..........................where babies like to sit
5.  Loaf................................. of bread | loaf................................................do nothing
6.  Land ............................... soil | land.........................put airplane on ground
7.  Log............................ships record | log...........................trunk of a tree
8.  Link .........................part of a chain | link......................................cuff links
9.  Left................................. remainder | left........................................ opposite of right
10. Limb ..........................tree branch | limb .........................part of the body
11. Lace ...........................crochet piece | lace......................................shoe tie
12. Lead......................... direct | lead .................................. head of a parade
13. Level .............................. even | level........................top story as in a house
14. Lord............................a ruler | lord ................................domineer, control
15. Leaf................part of a tree | leaf.......................................pages in a book
16. Last...........................endure | last........................................... final
17. Lodge......................place to stay | lodge............................................organization

# WORDS USED TWO WAYS - SOME ARE SLANG 11

CREATED BY GLENN SEYMOUR

1.    Mug _____    mug _____

2.    Mix _____    mix _____

3.    Mack _____    mack _____

4.    Map _____    map _____

5.    Mule _____    mule _____

6.    Mark _____    mark _____

7.    Mine _____    mine _____

8.    Mold _____    mold _____

9.    Mop _____    mop _____

10.   Match _____    match _____

11.   Mat _____    mat _____

12.   Mole _____    mole _____

13.   Mouse _____    mouse _____

14.   Mind _____    mind _____

15.   Mist _____    mist _____

16.   Mite _____    mite _____

17.   Note _____    note _____

# WORDS USED TWO WAYS - SOME ARE SLANG 11
## CREATED BY GLENN SEYMOUR

1. Mug ................................cup     mug ............................................ face
2. Mix .............................. mingle     mix............................................ stir
3. Mack............................. truck     mack.........................McDonald sandwich
4. Map ...............................atlas     map...........................lay out as a route
5. Mule ......................... animal     mule.......................................... shoe
6. Mark...............................brand     mark ................................... point out
7. Mine...........................ore deposit     mine ............................belonging to me
8. Mold............................to shape     mold ................................... to spoil
9. Mop .............................scrub     mop ...................... thick head of hair
10. Match ........................ alike     match..........................used to light a fire
11. Mat .............................. rug     mat........................... tangled mess
12. Mole ...........................rodent     mole............................... birthmark
13. Mouse..........................rodent     mouse...................... used with computer
14. Mind...........................obey     mind........................................brain
15. Mist ..............................fog     mist............................spray lightly
16. Mite ............................bug     mite................................ small amount
17. Note.............................reminder     note...........................musical writing

# WORDS USED TWO WAYS - SOME ARE SLANG 12

## CREATED BY GLENN SEYMOUR

1.   Navy _____          Navy _____

2.   Net_____            net_____

3.   Name_____           name_____

4.   Nag _____           nag _____

5.   Nap _____           nap _____

6.   Nut _____           nut _____

7.   Nick_____           nick_____

8.   Nutty_____          nutty_____

9.   Over _____          over_____

10.  Organ _____         organ_____

11.  Order_____          order_____

12.  Open _____          open _____

13.  Oath _____          oath_____

14.  Orange_____         orange_____

15.  Out _____           out_____

16.  Odd_____            odd _____

17.  Object _____        object _____

# WORDS USED TWO WAYS - SOME ARE SLANG 12
## CREATED BY GLENN SEYMOUR

1. Navy ..................... color                navy ..................... branch of service
2. Net ..................... trap                 net ..................... keep fish in
3. Name ..................... title               name ..................... point out
4. Nag ..................... torment              nag ..................... old horse
5. Nap ..................... short sleep          nap ..................... pile of carpet
6. Nut ..................... acorn                nut ..................... part of a bolt
7. Nick ..................... mar                 nick ..................... full of old nick
8. Nutty ..................... flavor             nutty ..................... whacky person
9. Over ..................... above               over ..................... the end of something
10. Organ ..................... part of the body  organ ..................... musical instrument
11. Order ..................... command           order ..................... supply of groceries
12. Open ..................... outspoken          open ..................... not shut
13. Oath ..................... pledge             oath ..................... sworn word
14. Orange ..................... fruit            orange ..................... color
15. Out ..................... not in              out ..................... not working
16. Odd ..................... different           odd ..................... not even
17. Object ..................... against - oppose object ..................... a thing - item

# WORDS USED TWO WAYS - SOME ARE SLANG 13
CREATED BY GLENN SEYMOUR

1.  Offer _____     offer _____

2.  Plug _____     plug _____

3.  Pad _____     pad _____

4.  Post _____     post _____

5.  Pit _____     pit _____

6.  Part _____     part _____

7.  Prune _____     prune _____

8.  Pen _____     pen _____

9.  Page _____     page _____

10. Pan _____     pan _____

11. Prop _____     prop _____

12. Park _____     park _____

13. Plot _____     plot _____

14. Print _____     print _____

15. Pine _____     pine _____

16. Pelt _____     pelt _____

17. Quiz _____     quiz _____

18. Quote _____     quote _____

# WORDS USED TWO WAYS - SOME ARE SLANG 13
## CREATED BY GLENN SEYMOUR

1. Offer ................... bid at an auction         offer ................................. volunteer

2. Plug ...................... stopper                 plug............................ speak out

3. Pad...................living quarters               pad........................ paper to write upon

4. Post.....................fence supporter            post.................... bring up to date

5. Pit ...............................hole             pit.............................cherry seed

6. Part ..........................separate             part ............................ section of a story

7. Prune.............................trim              prune..............................dried fruit

8. Pen................. writing instrument             pen..............................an enclosure

9. Page ...............leaf in a book                  page ......................... call a person

10. Pan..............................pot               pan..............................look for gold

11. Prop......................support                  prop .............. articles used in a stage show

12. Park ......................... resort              park ...........................gear in a car

13. Plot ......................... scheme              plot...........................garden spot

14. Print ..................... form of writing         print.........................................copy

15. Pine.............................tree              pine................................mourn

16. Pelt......................hit or strike            pelt.............................. animal hide

17. Quiz.................. question a person            quiz.........................test in school

18. Quote ...................... recite poetry          quote...................give an estimate on a job

# WORDS USED TWO WAYS - SOME ARE SLANG 14

CREATED BY GLENN SEYMOUR

1.  Quack _____ quack _____

2.  Quiver _____ quiver _____

3.  Quarter _____ quarter _____

4.  Quill _____ quill _____

5.  Queen _____ queen _____

6.  Rat _____ rat _____

7.  Ram _____ ram _____

8.  Rut _____ rut _____

9.  Rug _____ rug _____

10. Rod _____ rod _____

11. Rack _____ rack _____

12. Race _____ race _____

13. Rock _____ rock _____

14. Ring _____ ring _____

15. Rail _____ rail _____

16. Ruler _____ ruler _____

17. Raft _____ raft _____

# WORDS USED TWO WAYS - SOME ARE SLANG 14
## CREATED BY GLENN SEYMOUR

1.  Quack.............................duck sound — quack............................... fake doctor
2.  Quiver ................................. shake — quiver .........................place to put arrows
3.  Quarter .............................coin — quarter..................................... place to live
4.  Quill .............................pen — quill...................................................feather
5.  Queen.............................ruler — queen.............................in a deck of cards
6.  Rat .............................rodent — rat.................................................inform - tell
7.  Ram .................................. butt — ram ...................................male sheep
8.  Rut ......................... dent in the road — rut ............................... repeat over and over
9.  Rug ......................... floor cover — rug ................................... hair piece
10. Rod .............................fishing pole — rod ............................... measure
11. Rack.............................antlers — rack................................... place to put guns
12. Race.............................contest — race .........................................class of people
13. Rock .............................. stone — rock.........................back & forth in a chair
14. Ring.............................jewelry — ring ................................. square for boxing
15. Rail .............................railroad track — rail.........................................................bird
16. Ruler.....................measuring piece — ruler............................... king - queen
17. Raft ...........................floating vessel — raft .........................................a large number

# WORDS USED TWO WAYS - SOME ARE SLANG 15
### CREATED BY GLENN SEYMOUR

1. Run _____ run _____

2. Rib _____ rib _____

3. Raid _____ raid _____

4. Root _____ root _____

5. Saw _____ saw _____

6. Star _____ star _____

7. Sash _____ sash _____

8. Slug _____ slug _____

9. Spring _____ spring _____

10. Sink _____ sink _____

11. Stack _____ stack _____

12. Strike _____ strike _____

13. Storm _____ storm _____

14. Stand _____ stand _____

15. Stoop _____ stoop _____

16. Snuff _____ snuff _____

17. Stick _____ stick _____

# WORDS USED TWO WAYS - SOME ARE SLANG 15
## CREATED BY GLENN SEYMOUR

1. Run ......................travel fast on foot — run ...................................... seek office

2. Rib ......................bone in the body — rib ...........................................torment - tease

3. Raid ......................insect spray — raid .........................................investigation

4. Root......................tree life - support — root ...........get to the bottom of a problem

5. Saw ........................................... seeing — saw........................................... tool

6. Star ........................ heavenly body — star ...........................leading role in a show

7. Sash ......................part of a window — sash....................................ladies belt

8. Slug........................... fake coin — slug .......................................... hit

9. Spring......................season — spring .....................................leap

10. Sink......................... basin in house — sink..................................ground settlement

11. Stack.............................pile — stack......................... pipe smoke comes out

12. Strike..............................hit — strike......................workers refuse to work

13. Storm.............................. weather — storm ............................ attack on someone

14. Stand ...................piece of furniture — stand.......................................remain erect

15. Stoop ....................... bend the body — stoop.................................... poach

16. Snuff...........................put out a fire — snuff................................. tobacco

17. Stick...............................twig — stick ...............................adhere to

# WORDS USED TWO WAYS - SOME ARE SLANG 16
## CREATED BY GLENN SEYMOUR

1.  Stump _____    Stump _____

2.  Sap _____    Sap _____

3.  Stain _____    Stain _____

4.  Trip _____    Trip _____

5.  Tongue _____    Tongue _____

6.  Table _____    table _____

7.  Tank _____    tank _____

8.  Trunk _____    trunk _____

9.  Tug _____    tug _____

10.  Trail _____    trail _____

11.  Total _____    total _____

12.  Tree _____    tree _____

13.  Tape _____    tape _____

14.  Tick _____    tick _____

15.  Tart _____    tart _____

16.  Tire _____    tire _____

17.  Train _____    train _____

# WORDS USED TWO WAYS - SOME ARE SLANG 16
## CREATED BY GLENN SEYMOUR

1. Stump..........................base of a tree        stump .......................................unable to act

2. Sap ........................... tree liquid        sap...............................takes ones strength

3. Stain...........................change color        stain ........................................................soil

4. Trip......................................journey        trip..................................................to set off

5. Tongue .............. part of the mouth        tongue .................................part of a wagon

6. Table...................piece of furniture        table...................contents in front of book

7. Tank...............vessel to store liquid        tank...........................................army vehicle

8. Trunk ..............Place to store items        trunk.........................................part of a tree

9. Tug...................................pull        tug......................................part of a harness

10. Trail .........................follow        trail ...........................riding - walking path

11. Total ...............................add        total.........................................whole - entire

12. Tree.............................woody plant        tree.......................corner someone or thing

13. Tape ...................measuring device        tape ............................. woven strip of cloth

14. Tick...................................bug        tick..........................................sound of a clock

15. Tart ....................................sour        tart ................................................a small pie

16. Tire ...........................grow weary        tire...........................................wheel on a car

17. Train ...........................locomotive        train .......................................................teach

# WORDS USED TWO WAYS - SOME ARE SLANG 17
## CREATED BY GLENN SEYMOUR

1.  Warp _____    warp _____

2.  Wave _____    wave _____

3.  Will _____    will _____

4.  Well _____    well _____

5.  Walk _____    walk _____

6.  Wage _____    wage _____

7.  Wire_____    wire_____

8.  Web _____    web _____

9.  Whip _____    whip _____

10. Watch _____    watch _____

11. Wolf_____    wolf_____

12. Wind _____    wind _____

13. Yen_____    yen _____

14. Yale _____    yale _____

15. Yard _____    yard_____

16. Yarn_____    yarn_____

17. Yellow _____    yellow _____

18. Yield _____    yield _____

19. Yak_____    yak _____

20. Zero_____    zero _____

21. Zone _____    zone _____

# WORDS USED TWO WAYS - SOME ARE SLANG 17
## CREATED BY GLENN SEYMOUR

| | | | |
|---|---|---|---|
| 1. | Warp.................beat - whip | warp................bent out of shape |
| 2. | Wave.................move hand | wave................water movement |
| 3. | Will.................desire to do well | will.............document dividing an estate |
| 4. | Well.................healthy | well................place to obtain water |
| 5. | Walk.................step | walk................narrow path |
| 6. | Wage.................salary | wage................start a war |
| 7. | Wire.................metal cord | wire................send a message |
| 8. | Web.................net - material | web................what a spider weaves |
| 9. | Whip.................mix - stir | whip................beat a person |
| 10. | Watch.................time piece | watch................look |
| 11. | Wolf.................animal | wolf................gobble down food |
| 12. | Wind.................air movement | wind................breeze |
| 13. | Yen.................money | yen................desire |
| 14. | Yale.................College | yale................lock |
| 15. | Yard.................grounds | yard................measure |
| 16. | Yarn.................tall tale | yarn................wool cord |
| 17. | Yellow.................color | yellow................cowardly |
| 18. | Yield.................give | yield................how much a crop yields |
| 19. | Yak.................talk | yak................animal |
| 20. | Zero.................nothing | zero................land on a target |
| 21. | Zone.................parking area | zone................time areas |

# OPPOSITES - 1
CREATED BY GLENN SEYMOUR

1. Old _____

2. Black _____

3. Large _____

4. Big _____

5. Raw _____

6. Fat _____

7. Rich _____

8. Wide _____

9. Heavy _____

10. Tall _____

11. Deep _____

12. Dim _____

13. Oral _____

14. Thin _____

15. Bad _____

16. Windy _____

17. Arid _____

18. Bold _____

19. Happy _____

20. Bitter _____

21. Busy _____

22. Edge _____

23. Back _____

24. Exit _____

25. Even _____

26. To _____

27. Ever _____

28. For _____

29. Few _____

30. Frown _____

31. Fast _____

32. Here _____

33. Kind _____

34. Long _____

35. Friend _____

36. Gain _____

# OPPOSITES - 1
CREATED BY GLENN SEYMOUR

1.  Old...................................... young
2.  Black......................................white
3.  Large...................................... small
4.  Big......................................little
5.  Raw......................................cooked
6.  Fat......................................slim
7.  Rich......................................poor
8.  Wide......................................narrow
9.  Heavy...................................... light
10. Tall...................................... short
11. Deep...................................... shallow
12. Dim......................................bright
13. Oral......................................written
14. Thin...................................... thick
15. Bad...................................... good
16. Windy......................................calm
17. Arid...................................... wet
18. Bold......................................timid

19. Happy...................................... sad
20. Bitter......................................sweet
21. Busy......................................idle
22. Edge......................................center
23. Back......................................front
24. Exit...................................... enter
25. Even...................................... odd
26. To......................................fro
27. Ever......................................ever
28. For......................................against
29. Few......................................many
30. Frown...................................... smile
31. Fast...................................... slow
32. Here...................................... there
33. Kind......................................mean
34. Long...................................... short
35. Friend......................................stranger
36. Gain......................................lose

# OPPOSITIES - 2
## CREATED BY GLENN SEYMOUR

1. Here _____

2. Under _____

3. Wrong_____

4. Frigid _____

5. Up_____

6. Coarse _____

7. Rough_____

8. Solid _____

9. Hard _____

10. Cloudy _____

11. Thick_____

12. Rainy _____

13. Wet_____

14. Shallow_____

15. Round_____

16. Love _____

17. Wild _____

18. Elevate _____

19. End_____

20. Difficult _____

21. Double _____

22. Correct_____

23. Do_____

24. Left_____

25. Top _____

26. Fix _____

27. Fib _____

28. Polished _____

29. Find _____

30. Go_____

31. Give _____

32. Succeed_____

33. Zig _____

34. Sit _____

35. Forget _____

36. Sure _____

# OPPOSITES - 2
## CREATED BY GLENN SEYMOUR

1. Here ............................................... there
2. Under ...........................................over
3. Wrong...........................................right
4. Frigid ..........................................hot
5. Up ............................................... down
6. Coarse .........................................fine
7. Rough...........................................smooth
8. Solid.............................................liquid
9. Hard.............................................soft
10. Cloudy..........................................clear
11. Thick............................................thin
12. Rainy ...........................................sunny
13. Wet..............................................dry
14. Shallow.........................................deep
15. Round...........................................square
16. Love ............................................hate
17. Wild.............................................tame
18. Elevate .........................................lower

19. End ...............................................begin
20. Difficult .......................................easy
21. Double..........................................single
22. Correct .........................................wrong
23. Do ...............................................don't
24. Left..............................................right
25. Top..............................................bottom
26. Fix ..............................................break
27. Fib .............................................. truth
28. Polished........................................dull
29. Find .............................................lose
30. Go ...............................................come
31. Give.............................................take
32. Succeed.........................................fail
33. Zig..............................................zag
34. Sit...............................................stand
35. Forget ..........................................remember
36. Sure............................................ doubtful

# EXPRESSIONS 1
CREATED BY GLENN SEYMOUR

1. He was so crooked.............................................................................................................
2. If looks could kill.............................................................................................................
3. Out of the frying pan.........................................................................................................
4. That farm is so poor.........................................................................................................
5. From a little acorn............................................................................................................
6. All that goes up.................................................................................................................
7. Two wrongs do not...........................................................................................................
8. Let it go in one ear...........................................................................................................
9. Never let your left hand....................................................................................................
10. Eat your..........................................................................................................................
11. Weigh your words...........................................................................................................
12. All work and no play.......................................................................................................
13. Now that's a horse...........................................................................................................
14. A penny for.....................................................................................................................
15. A fool and his money......................................................................................................
16. He has one foot in the grave and.....................................................................................
17. He is not worth...............................................................................................................
18. Let sleeping dogs............................................................................................................
19. All is well that................................................................................................................
20. Judge not lest.................................................................................................................
21. His bark is worse than.....................................................................................................
22. Like paying for a.............................................................................................................
23. People who live in glass houses.......................................................................................
24. Just missed by a..............................................................................................................
25. He just sat there like.......................................................................................................
26. Close only counts in........................................................................................................
27. That is the way the cookie...............................................................................................
28. Don't leave any stone......................................................................................................
29. Invention is the result......................................................................................................
30. Strike while the...............................................................................................................
31. That was a close.............................................................................................................

# EXPRESSIONS 1
## CREATED BY GLENN SEYMOUR

1. He was so crooked ........................................................ he couldn't lay straight
2. If looks could kill ............................................................. I would be dead
3. Out of the frying pan ........................................................ into the fire
4. That farm is so poor ................................................ you couldn't raise a fuss on it
5. From a little acorn ........................................................ grows a mighty oak tree
6. All that goes up .............................................................. must come down
7. Two wrongs do not ........................................................... make a right
8. Let it go in one ear .......................................................... and out another
9. Never let your left hand ........................................ know what the right hand is doing
10. Eat your ........................................................................ heart out
11. Weigh your words ............................................................. before you speak
12. All work and no play .................................................... makes Jack a dull boy
13. Now that's a horse ........................................................ of a different color
14. A penny for ..................................................................... your thoughts
15. A fool and his money ........................................................ are soon parted
16. He had one foot in the grave .............................. an another on a banana peel
17. He is not worth ................................................. the powder and lead to blow him up
18. Let sleeping dogs ........................................................................... lie
19. All is well that ..................................................................... ends well
20. Judge not less ..................................................................... you be judged
21. His bark is worse than his ..................................................... bite
22. Like paying for a ............................................................. dead horse
23. People who live in glass houses .......................... should throw stones
24. Just missed by .................................................................. by a hair
25. He just sat there like a .................................................... bump on a log
26. Close only counts in .......................................................... horseshoes
27. That is the way the cookie ................................................ crumbles
28. Don't leave any stone ........................................................ unturned
29. Invention is the result ........................................................ of necessity
30. Strike while the ................................................................ iron is hot
31. That was a close .................................................................... call

212

# EXPRESSIONS 2
## CREATED BY GLENN SEYMOUR

1. Jump right in and ......................................................................

2. You must learn to crawl ..............................................................

3. He moves as slow as ...................................................................

4. She has the patience of................................................................

5. He is skating on ........................................................................

6. About four miles as ....................................................................

7. Just a drop in the ......................................................................

8. Hitch your wagon........................................................................

9. He is the talk of........................................................................

10. He is higher than a .....................................................................

11. I'm weaker than a .......................................................................

12. He delivered his speech ...............................................................

13. He is talking .............................................................................

14. He gave an answer without .............................................................

15. Not worth a ..............................................................................

16. It is darkest just before................................................................

17. Take the bull..............................................................................

18. Fly off the handle........................................................................

19. I don't trust him any farther than I can................................................

20. Sticks & stones may break my back but.................................................

21. Whistling girls and crowing hens......................................................

22. Believe none of what you hear and ....................................................

# EXPRESSIONS 2
## CREATED BY GLENN SEYMOUR

1.  Jump right in and ................................................................ get your feet wet

2.  You must learn to crawl ..................................................... before you walk

3.  He moves as slow as a ................................................................... snail

4.  She has the patience of ..................................................................... job

5.  He is skating on ...................................................................... thin ice

6.  About four miles as the ............................................................. crow flics

7.  Just a drop in the .................................................................... bucket

8.  Hitch your wagon ................................................................. to a star

9.  He is the talk of the .................................................................. town

10. He is higher than a ...................................................................... kite

11. I'm weaker than a ...................................................................... cat

12. He delivered his speech ...................................................... right off the cuff

13. He is talking ................................................................ through his hat

14. He gave an answer without ................................................. blinking an eye

15. Not worth a .......................................................................... red cent

16. It is darkest just before ............................................................. the dawn

17. Take the bull ........................................................................ by his horns

18. Fly off the handle ..................................................................... get mad

19. I don't trust him any farther than I can ....................... throw a bull by his horns

20. Stick & stones may break my back but .................. words will never harm me

21. Whistling girls and crowing hens ............................... often come to a bad end

22. Believe none of what you hear and ........................ only half of what you see

# ANOTHER NAME
## CREATED BY GLENN SEYMOUR

1.  Ebb .................................................................................................................
2.  Summit ............................................................................................................
3.  Gap ..................................................................................................................
4.  Median ............................................................................................................
5.  Arc ..................................................................................................................
6.  Triangle ...........................................................................................................
7.  Campus ...........................................................................................................
8.  Junker .............................................................................................................
9.  Square .............................................................................................................
10. Cab .................................................................................................................
11. Cane ................................................................................................................
12. Nag .................................................................................................................
13. Cur .................................................................................................................
14. Burro ..............................................................................................................
15. Prince Albert ...................................................................................................
16. Hobo ..............................................................................................................
17. Sturgeon .........................................................................................................
18. Packadurm .......................................................................................................
19. Vixen ..............................................................................................................
20. Dorm ..............................................................................................................
21. Yardstick .........................................................................................................
22. Dinghy ............................................................................................................
23. Maiden Blush ...................................................................................................
24. Tumbler ..........................................................................................................
25. Cartwheel ........................................................................................................

# ANOTHER NAME
## CREATED BY GLENN SEYMOUR

1. Ebb ................................................................................ low tide

2. Summit ....................................................... top - peak

3. Gap .............................................. a break in something

4. Median ....................................grass strip between a divided highway

5. Arc .................................................... part of a circle

6. Triangle ..............................................three sided figure

7. Campus.......................................... College grounds

8. Junker ..............................................................old car

9. Square ...................................four sides - equal length

10. Cab ....................................................................taxi

11. Cane ........................................................ walking stick

12. Nag ..........................................................old horse

13. Cur................................................................ dog

14. Burro .............................................small donkey

15. Prince Albert.......................................... smoking tobacco

16. Hobo .................................................... tramp

17. Sturgeon...................................................fish

18. Packadurm .......................................... elephant

19. Vixen .......................................................fox

20. Dorm..........................................College living quarters

21. Yard stick ..................................three foot measuring tool

22. Dinghy .................................................. boat

23. Maiden Blush ......................................apple

24. Tumbler ....................................... drinking glass

25. Cartwheel ........................................ silver dollar

# ABREVATIONS 1
CREATED BY GLENN SEYMOUR

1.  AAA ....................................................................................................................................

2.  ACCT ..................................................................................................................................

3.  BLDG ..................................................................................................................................

4.  BRO .....................................................................................................................................

5.  CCC .....................................................................................................................................

6.  CHEM ................................................................................................................................

7.  DAR .....................................................................................................................................

8.  DEG .....................................................................................................................................

9.  EKG .....................................................................................................................................

10. ELEM ..................................................................................................................................

11. FBI .......................................................................................................................................

12. FCC ......................................................................................................................................

13. GAL ......................................................................................................................................

14. GEN .....................................................................................................................................

15. HGT .....................................................................................................................................

16. HOSP ..................................................................................................................................

17. IOOF ...................................................................................................................................

18. IOV ......................................................................................................................................

19. LAB ......................................................................................................................................

20. LBS ......................................................................................................................................

21. MED .....................................................................................................................................

22. MFG .....................................................................................................................................

23. NBA .....................................................................................................................................

24. NBC .....................................................................................................................................

25. OBJ ......................................................................................................................................

26. OBIT ...................................................................................................................................

27. PCT ......................................................................................................................................

28. PER ......................................................................................................................................

29. RBI .......................................................................................................................................

30. RAF ......................................................................................................................................

# ABBREVIATIONS 1
## CREATED BY GLENN SEYMOUR

1. AAA ............................................................................ American Automobile Association
2. Acct ............................................................................................................ account
3. Bldg ........................................................................................................... building
4. Bro ............................................................................................................... brother
5. CCC ........................................................................ Civilian Conservation Corporation
6. Chem ........................................................................................................ chemistry
7. DAR ........................................................................ Daughters of the American Revolution
8. Deg ............................................................................................................... degree
9. EKG ................................................................................................ electric Cardiogram
10. Elem ....................................................................................................... elementary
11. FBI ....................................................................................... Federal Bureau of Investigation
12. FCC ...................................................................... Federal Communication Commission
13. Gal ............................................................................................................. gallon
14. Gen ........................................................................................................... General
15. Hgt .............................................................................................................. height
16. Hosp .......................................................................................................... Hospital
17. IOOF ........................................................................ Independent Order of Odd Fellows
18. IOV ........................................................................................................... I love you
19. Lab ........................................................................................................... labatory
20. Lbs ............................................................................................................. pounds
21. Med ........................................................................................................... medical
22. Mfg .......................................................................................................... manufacture
23. NBA ...................................................................................... National Basketball Association
24. NBC ...................................................................................... National Broadcasting Commission
25. Obj .............................................................................................................. object
26. Obit ........................................................................................................... obituary
27. Pct .............................................................................................................. percent
28. Per .............................................................................................................. person
29. RBI ........................................................................................................ runs batted in
30. RAF ........................................................................................................ Royal Air Force

# ABBREVIATIONS 2
CREATED BY GLENN SEYMOUR

1.  HWY ............................................................................................................

2.  IRS .............................................................................................................

3.  INT .............................................................................................................

4.  LGE ............................................................................................................

5.  LTD .............................................................................................................

6.  LGT .............................................................................................................

7.  MIL .............................................................................................................

8.  MPH ............................................................................................................

9.  NEG .............................................................................................................

10. NRA .............................................................................................................

11. NUM ............................................................................................................

12. PD ...............................................................................................................

13. POW ............................................................................................................

14. REG .............................................................................................................

15. REF .............................................................................................................

16. SECY ...........................................................................................................

17. SEN .............................................................................................................

18. TKO .............................................................................................................

19. USA .............................................................................................................

20. USPS ...........................................................................................................

21. VOL .............................................................................................................

22. YMCA ..........................................................................................................

23. YWCA ..........................................................................................................

24. AFL .............................................................................................................

25. AMT ............................................................................................................

26. CPA .............................................................................................................

# ABBREVATIONS 2
CREATED BY GLENN SEYMOUR

1. HWY .............................................................................................HIGHWAY
2. IRS ..................................................................... INTERNAL REVENUE SERVICE
3. INT ...............................................................................................INTEREST
4. LGE ................................................................................................ LARGE
5. LTD ............................................................................................. LIMITED
6. LGT ..................................................................................................LIGHT
7. MIL ...............................................................................MILLION - MILITARY
8. MPH ............................................................................... MILE PER HOUR
9. NEG .............................................................................................NEGATIVE
10. NRA ..................................................................NATIONAL RIFLE ASSOCIATION
11. NUM ............................................................................................NUMBER
12. PD ..................................................................................................... PAID
13.. POW ..................................................................................PRISONER OF WAR
14. REG .............................................................................................. REGULAR
15. REF ............................................................................................... REFEREE
16. SECY .........................................................................................SECRETARY
17. SEN............................................................................................... SENATOR
18. TKO.................................................................................TECHINAL KNOCK OUT
19. USA .............................................................. UNITED STATE OF AMERICA
20. USPS..............................................................UNITED STATES POSTAL SERVICE
21. VOL .............................................................................................. VOLUME
22. YMCA ......................................................... YOUNG MENS CHRISTIAN ASSOCIATION
23. YWCA .....................................................YOUNG WOMENS CHRISTIAN ASSOCIATION
24. AFL................................................................ AMERICAN FEDERATION OF LABOR
25. AMT ...............................................................................................AMOUNT
26. CPA ........................................................... CERTIFIED PUBLIC ACCOUNTANT

# LITTLE THINGS TO PONDER
CREATED BY GLENN SEYMOUR

1. Peach _____
2. Bull _____
3. Goose _____
4. Ram _____
5. Whip _____
6. Pork _____
7. Electric _____
8. Icy _____
9. Dogwood _____
10. Horse _____
11. Pony _____
12. Cotton _____
13. Bull _____
14. Mud _____
15. Sink _____
16. Back _____
17. Ice _____
18. Lead _____
19. Gold _____
20. Marble _____
21. Saw _____

22. Butter _____
23. Cat _____
24. Ham _____
25. Fox _____
26. Buffalo _____
27. Crab _____
28. Scotch _____
29. Honey _____
30. Coffee _____
31. Turkish _____
32. Witch _____
33. Mush _____
34. Cat _____
35. Butter _____
36. Tea _____
37. Babies _____
38. Steel _____
39. Stool _____
40. Eskimo _____
41. Car _____
42. Ivory _____

# LITTLE THINGS TO PONDER
## CREATED BY GLENN SEYMOUR

1. Peach ..................................... cobbler
2. Bull..............................................horn
3. Goose ...................................... bumps
4. Ram ............................................. rod
5. Whip.......................................... lash
6. Pork ....................................... barrel
7. Electric .....................................eel
8. Icy ...............................................hot
9. Dogwood ...............................tree
10. Horse ................................... radish
11. Pony.........................................tail
12. Cotton .................................candy
13. Bull.......................................dozer
14. Mud .....................................dobber
15. Sink........................................hole
16. Back .........................................log
17. Ice............................................cube
18. Lead ......................................pencil
19. Gold....................................... digger
20. Marble ................................cake
21. Saw..........................................horse

22. Butter...............................bean
23. Cat.........................................nip
24. Ham..................................burger
25. Fox ........................................ glove
26. Buffalo ............................ wings
27. Crab ..................................... apple
28. Scotch .................................tape
29. Honey................................. dew
30. Coffee ...................................cake
31. Turkish ...............................towel
32. Witch .................................. hazel
33. Mush.................................room
34. Cat.........................................tail
35. Butter.......................................fly
36. Tea........................................kettle
37. Babies ...................................breath
38. Steel ......................................wool
39. Stool.................................. pigeon
40. Eskimo ..............................pie
41. Car .......................................... pool
42. Ivory ....................................... soap

222

# ANOTHER NAME
## CREATED BY GLENN SEYMOUR

1.  Cartwheel .......................................................................................................................
2.  Cockscomb .......................................................................................................................
3.  Lea .......................................................................................................................
4.  Lei .......................................................................................................................
5.  Whippet .......................................................................................................................
6.  Alumni .......................................................................................................................
7.  Gillette .......................................................................................................................
8.  Know hole .......................................................................................................................
9.  Bogus check .......................................................................................................................
10. Honey dew .......................................................................................................................
11. Firmament .......................................................................................................................
12. El .......................................................................................................................
13. Killdeer .......................................................................................................................
14. Catamaran .......................................................................................................................
15. R.N. .......................................................................................................................
16. Mae West .......................................................................................................................
17. Merry Go Round .......................................................................................................................
18. Group of Stores .......................................................................................................................
19. Yellow flashing light .......................................................................................................................
20. Red flashing light .......................................................................................................................
21. Spreading Viper .......................................................................................................................
22. Stopwatch .......................................................................................................................
23. Bittersweet .......................................................................................................................
24. Dromedary .......................................................................................................................
25. Essex .......................................................................................................................
26. Textbooks .......................................................................................................................

# ANOTHER NAME
## CREATED BY GLENN SEYMOUR

1.  Cartwheel ...................................................................... silver dollar

2.  Cockscomb ........................................................................... flower

3.  Lea ...................................................................... meadow - pasture

4.  Lei ..................................................... necklace made of flowers

5.  Whippet ....................................................................... racing dog

6.  Alumni ................................................................. school graduate

7.  Gillette ..................................................................................... razor

8.  Knot hole ...................................hole where a piece of wood fell out

9.  Bogus check ........................................ check with no funds to cover it

10. Honey Dew ........................................................................... melon

11. Firmament .................................................................................. sky

12. El ........................................................................ elevated highway

13. Killdeer ...................................................................................... bird

14. Catamaran ...................................................................... raft - float

15. R.N ....................................................................... registered nurse

16. Mae West ............................................................... life jacket

17. Merry go round .................................................................. carousal

18. Group of stores ..................................................................... mall

19. Yellow flashing light .......................................................... warning

20. Red flashing light ................................................................... stop

21. Spreading viper ................................................................... snake

22. Stopwatch ................................................................. timing device

23. Bittersweet ........................................................ shrub with berries

24. Dromedary ....................................................................... camel

25. Essex .......................................................................................... car

26. Textbooks ..................................................................... school books

# CALENDAR
## CREATED BY GLENN SEYMOUR

1.  What is January 1st? ..........................................................................
2.  What is January 15th? .......................................................................
3.  When is Groundhog Day? ...................................................................
4.  When is Lincoln's birthday? ...............................................................
5.  What is February 15th? ......................................................................
6.  February 19th is? ..............................................................................
7.  Whose birthday is February 22nd? ......................................................
8.  When is St. Patrick's day? ..................................................................
9.  April 1st is? ......................................................................................
10. May 1st brings? .................................................................................
11. Some Sunday in April is? ....................................................................
12. April 15th you pay your? .....................................................................
13. What parent has a special day in May? .................................................
14. May 30th is? ......................................................................................
15. June 14th is? ......................................................................................
16. A special parent day in June is? ...........................................................
17. July 4th is? ........................................................................................
18. What are the days in August called? ....................................................
19. First Monday in September is? .............................................................
20. October 12th is? ................................................................................
21. Halloween is what day? ......................................................................
22. When is Election Day? .......................................................................
23. When is Veteran's Day? ......................................................................
24. Thanksgiving Day is? .........................................................................
25. What is December 7th? .......................................................................
26. When is Christmas? ...........................................................................

# CALENDAR
## CREATED BY GLENN SEYMOUR

1.  What is January 1st? ....................................................................New Years Day

2.  What is January 15th? ..................................Martin Luther Kings birthday

3.  When is Groundhog Day? ..................................................... February 2nd

4.  When is Lincoln's birthday? ............................................... February 12th

5.  What is February 14th? ......................................................Valentines Day

6.  February 19th is? ....................................................................Presidents Day

7.  Whose birthday is February 22nd? ................................ George Washington

8.  When is St. Patrick's day? ..................................................... March 17th

9.  April 1st is? .................................................................... April's Fools Day

10. May 1st brings? ...................................................................... May flowers

11. Some Sunday in April is? .................................................... .......Easter

12. April 15th you pay your? ................................................................. taxes

13. What parent has a special day in May? ...................................Mother's Day

14. May 30th is? ......................................................................Memorial Day

15. June 14th is? ...................................................................................Flag Day

16. A special parent day in June is? .......................................Father's Day

17. July 4th is? ...................................................................Independence Day

18. What are the days in August called? ........................... Dog's Day of August

19. First Monday in September is? .................................................Labor Day

20. October 12th is? ...................................................................Columbus Day

21. Halloween day is what day? ..................................................October 31st

22. When is Election day? ........................... second Tuesday after first Monday

23. When is Veteran's Day? .................................................. November 11th

24. Thanksgiving Day is? ..............................fourth Thursday in November

25. What is December 7th? ................................................ .Pearl Harbor Day

26. When is Christmas? ..............................................................December 25th

# WORDS PRONOUNCED THE SAME
# SPELLED DIFFERENTLY
CREATED BY GLENN SEYMOUR

1. HEART _____

2. HOLE _____

3. HIGHER _____

4. HIGH _____

5. IN _____

6. ISLE _____

7. JEAN _____

8. HOES _____

9. KNEAD _____

10. JAM _____

11. KNEW _____

12. KNOT _____

13. LOAD _____

14. KNOW _____

15. LEAN _____

16. LONE _____

17. LESSON _____

18. LOOT _____

19. LIRE _____

20. LEAK _____

21. MALL _____

22. LACKS _____

23. MADE _____

24. MAIN _____

25. MEET _____

26. MAIL _____

27. NO _____

28. MIGHT _____

29. OLEO _____

30. MARRY _____

31. ONE _____

32. NUN _____

33. PAIN _____

34. OUR _____

35. PARE _____

36. PAIL _____

37. PUGH _____

38. PEALE _____

39. POOR _____

40. PEAK _____

41. PAUSE _____

42. PIE _____

43. QUART _____

44. QUAIL _____

# WORDS PRONOUNCED THE SAME
## SPELLED DIFFERENTLY
CREATED BY GLENN SEYMOUR

| | | | | | |
|---|---|---|---|---|---|
| 1. | HEART | HART | 23. | MADE | MAID |
| 2. | HOLE | WHOLE | 24. | MAIN | MANE |
| 3. | HIGHER | HIRE | 25. | MEET | MEAT |
| 4. | HIGH | HI | 26. | MAIL | MALE |
| 5. | IN | INN | 27. | NO | KNOW |
| 6. | ISLE | AISLE | 28. | MIGHT | MITE |
| 7. | JEAN | GENE | 29. | OLEO | OLIO |
| 8. | HOES | HOSE | 30. | MARRY | MERRY |
| 9. | KNEAD | NEED | 31. | ONE | WON |
| 10. | JAM | JAMB | 32. | NUN | NONE |
| 11. | KNEW | NEW | 33. | PAIN | PANE |
| 12. | KNOT | NOT | 34. | OUR | HOUR |
| 13. | LOAD | LODE | 35. | PARE | PAIR |
| 14. | KNOW | NO | 36. | PAIL | PALE |
| 15. | LEAN | LIEN | 37. | PUGH | PEW |
| 16. | LONE | LOAN | 38. | PEALE | PEEL |
| 17. | LESSON | LESSEN | 39. | POOR | POUR |
| 18. | LOOT | LUTE | 40. | PEAK | PEEK |
| 19. | LIRE | LYRE | 41. | PAUSE | PAWS |
| 20. | LEAK | LEEK | 42. | PIE | PI |
| 21. | MALL | MAUL | 43. | QUART | QUARTZ |
| 22. | LACKS | LAX | 44. | QUAIL | QUAYLE |

# MISSING WORDS
## CREATED BY GLENN SEYMOUR

1. Women's.................................................................................................

2. Rome wasn't built in a...........................................................................

3. Jack and................................................................................................

4. Bury the................................................................................................

5. Diamonds are a girls.............................................................................

6. Like paying for a...................................................................................

7. Honest...................................................................................................

8. OOHS and.............................................................................................

9. I could eat a..........................................................................................

10. The surrey with the fringe....................................................................

11. Shake a..................................................................................................

12. Fe Fi Fo.................................................................................................

13. Alice Blue..............................................................................................

14. Busy as a...............................................................................................

15. A partridge in a.....................................................................................

16. Carlsbad................................................................................................

17. Bric and.................................................................................................

18. Garden of..............................................................................................

19. Up a lazy................................................................................................

20. Feast of.................................................................................................

21. It's not worth a......................................................................................

22. If, ands, no butts...................................................................................

23. Low fat..................................................................................................

24. Up a lazy................................................................................................

25. Garden of..............................................................................................

# MISSING WORD
## CREATED BY GLENN SEYMOUR

1.  Women's .................................................................................................... lib

2.  Rome wasn't built in a .......................................................................... day

3.  Jack and ................................................................................................. Jill

4.  Bury the ............................................................................................ hatchet

5.  Diamonds are a girls ...................................................... best friend

6.  Like paying for a ........................................................................ dead horse

7.  Honest ................................................................................................... Abe

8.  OOHs and ......................................................................................... AAHS

9.  I could eat a .................................................................................... horse

10. The surrey with a ............................................................. fringe on top

11. Shake a .................................................................................................. leg

12. To and .................................................................................................. fro

13. FeFiFo ................................................................................................. Fum

14. Alice Blue .......................................................................................... gown

15. Busy as a .............................................................................................. bee

16. A partridge in a ........................................................................ pear tree

17. Carlsbad ...................................................................................... Caverns

18. Bric and ............................................................................................. brac

19. Feast or ........................................................................................... famine

20. It's not worth a .......................................................................... plug nickel

21. If, ands, no butts ...................................................................... about it

22. Low fat ................................................................................................ diet

23. Up a lazy .......................................................................................... river

24. Garden of ......................................................................................... Eden

# WHAT IS IT?
## CREATED BY GLENN SEYMOUR

1.  Essex......................................................................................................................

2.  Downy....................................................................................................................

3.  Ritz .......................................................................................................................

4.  Bic........................................................................................................................

5.  Lava.......................................................................................................................

6.  Evinrude.................................................................................................................

7.  Ocean Spray ...........................................................................................................

8.  Blackeyed...............................................................................................................

9.  Burpless .................................................................................................................

10. Tutu.......................................................................................................................

11. Tam.......................................................................................................................

12. Mini.......................................................................................................................

13. Baby Grand ............................................................................................................

14. Sunmaid.................................................................................................................

15. Arrow.....................................................................................................................

16. Timex.....................................................................................................................

17. Bunn......................................................................................................................

18. Seyelle ...................................................................................................................

19. Clydesdale ..............................................................................................................

20. Ball........................................................................................................................

21. McCormick .............................................................................................................

22. Goodyear................................................................................................................

23. Bosc ......................................................................................................................

24. Pippin.....................................................................................................................

# WHAT IS IT?
## CREATED BY GLENN SEYMOUR

1.  Essex .................................................................................................... car
2.  Downy ................................................................................... fabric softener
3.  Ritz ................................................................................................. cracker
4.  Bic ............................................................................................ fountain pen
5.  Lava ................................................................................................... soap
6.  Evinrude ......................................................................................... battery
7.  Ocean Spray ......................................................................... cranberry juice
8.  Blackeyed ........................................................................................... peas
9.  Burpless ...................................................................................... cucumber
10. Tutu ................................................................................................... skirt
11. Tam ......................................................................................... brimless cap
12. Mini ................................................................................................... skirt
13. Baby Grand ...................................................................................... piano
14. Sunmaid .......................................................................................... raisins
15. Arrow ................................................................................................ shirt
16. Timex ............................................................................................... watch
17. Bunn ...................................................................................... coffee maker
18. Seyelle ............................................................................................... yarn
19. Clydesdale ....................................................................................... horse
20. Ball ..................................................................................... canning supplies
21. McCormick ....................................................................................... spice
22. Goodyear ............................................................................................ tires
23. Bosc ................................................................................................... pear
24. Pippin ............................................................................................... apple

# WORDS SOUND SAME - SPELLED DIFFERENTLY 1

CREATED BY GLENN SEYMOUR

1. Heart _____

2. Read _____

3. Wright _____

4. Lean _____

5. Plain _____

6. Pray _____

7. Vale _____

8. Four _____

9. Fair _____

10. Sail _____

11. Sore _____

12. Tail _____

13. Led _____

14. Wrap _____

15. Ring _____

16. Route _____

17. Gate _____

18. Stair _____

19. Abel _____

20. Raise _____

21. Flu _____

22. Flee _____

23. Sum _____

24. Son _____

25. Seed _____

26. Bowl _____

27. Knew _____

28. Enter _____

29. Waist _____

30. Stayed _____

31. Site _____

32. Die _____

# WORDS SOUND SAME - SPELLED DIFFERENTLY 1

CREATED BY GLENN SEYMOUR

| | | | | |
|---|---|---|---|---|
| 1. | Heart | hart | 17. Gate | gait |
| 2. | Read | reed | 18. Stair | stare |
| 3. | Wright | right | 19. Abel | able |
| 4. | Lean | lien | 20. Raise | raze |
| 5. | Plain | plane | 21. Flu | flew |
| 6. | Pray | prey | 22. Flee | flea |
| 7. | Vale | veil | 23. Sum | some |
| 8. | Four | for | 24. Son | sun |
| 9. | Fair | fare | 25. Seed | cede |
| 10. | Sail | sale | 26. Bowl | bole |
| 11. | Sore | soar | 27. Knew | new |
| 12. | Tail | tale | 28. Enter | inter |
| 13. | Led | lead | 29. Waist | waste |
| 14. | Wrap | rap | 30. Stayed | staid |
| 15. | Ring | wring | 31. Site | sight |
| 16. | Route | rout | 32. Die | dye |

# WORDS SOUND SAME - SPELLED DIFFERENTLY 2
CREATED BY GLENN SEYMOUR

1. AID _____

2. ALL _____

3. ANT _____

4. AIL _____

5. ABLE _____

6. ARC _____

7. AIR _____

8. ATE _____

9. AISLE _____

10. BEAU _____

11. BREAK _____

12. BEAR _____

13. BE _____

14. BEAT _____

15. BLEW _____

16. BEEN _____

17. BURN _____

18. BOAR _____

19. BUT _____

20. BAIL _____

21. COAT _____

22. COAL _____

23. CENT _____

24. CITE _____

25. CELL _____

26. CRAFT _____

27. DOE _____

28. DEW _____

29. DISK _____

30. DEER _____

31. EAVE _____

32. EARN _____

33. EWE _____

34. FOUR _____

35. FLOW _____

36. FEET _____

37. FLEW _____

38. FLEE _____

39. GAIL _____

40. GRATE _____

41. GROAN _____

42. GATE _____

43. HOUR _____

44. HAIL _____

45. HAIR _____

46. HALL _____

# WORDS SOUND SAME - SPELLED DIFFERENTLY 2

CREATED BY GLENN SEYMOUR

1.   AID............................................... ade
2.   ALL............................................... awl
3.   ANT...............................................aunt
4.   AIL............................................... ale
5.   ABLE............................................... abel
6.   ARC...............................................ark
7.   AIR............................................... heir
8.   ATE...............................................eight
9.   AISLE ...............................................isle
10.  BEAU...............................................bow
11.  BREAK...............................................brake
12.  BEAR...............................................bare
13.  BE............................................... bee
14.  BEAT...............................................beet
15.  BLEW...............................................blue
16.  BEEN...............................................bin
17.  BURN...............................................Byrne
18.  BOAR............................................... bore
19.  BUT ............................................... butt
20.  BAIL...............................................bale
21.  COAT ...............................................cote
22.  COAL...............................................cole
23.  CENT ............................................... scent
24.  CITE...............................................sight
25.  CELL...............................................sell
26.  CRAFT...............................................kraft
27.  DOE...............................................dough
28.  DEW...............................................do - due
29.  DISK............................................... disc
30.  DEER...............................................dear
31.  EAVE...............................................eve
32.  EARN ...............................................urn
33.  EWE ...............................................you
34.  FOUR ............................................... fore
35.  FLOW...............................................floe
36.  FEET...............................................fete
37.  FLEW...............................................flue
38.  FLEE...............................................flea
39.  GAIL...............................................gale
40.  GRATE...............................................grate
41.  GROAN ...............................................grown
42.  GATE...............................................gait
43.  HOUR ............................................... our
44.  HAIL...............................................hale
45.  HAIR...............................................hare
46.  HALL...............................................haul